Integrating Exercise, Sports, Movement and Mind: Therapeutic Unity

Integrating Exercise, Sports, Movement and Mind: Therapeutic Unity has been co-published simultaneously as *The Psychotherapy Patient*, Volume 10, Numbers 3/4 1998.

Integrating Exercise, Sports, Movement and Mind: Therapeutic Unity

Kate F. Hays
Editor

E. Mark Stern
Series Editor

Integrating Exercise, Sports, Movement and Mind: Therapeutic Unity has been co-published simultaneously as *The Psychotherapy Patient*, Volume 10, Numbers 3/4 1998.

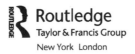

Routledge
Taylor & Francis Group
New York London

Integrating Exercise, Sports, Movement and Mind: Therapeutic Unity has been co-published simultaneously as *The Psychotherapy Patient*, Volume 10, Numbers 3/4 1998.

First published 1998 by The Haworth Press, Inc.

Published 2021 by Routledge
605 Third Avenue, New York, NY 10017
2 Park Square, Milton Park, Abingdon, Oxon OX14 4RN

Routledge is an imprint of the Taylor & Francis Group, an informa business

Cover design by Thomas J. Mayshock Jr.

Library of Congress Cataloging-in-Publication Data

Integrating exercise, sports, movement, and mind : therapeutic unity / Kate F. Hays, editor; E. Mark Stern, series editor.
   p. cm.
   Also published as The psychotherapy patient, v. 10, nos. 3/4, 1998.
   Includes bibliographical references and index.
   ISBN 0-7890-0380-5 (alk. paper). – ISBN 0-7890-0384-8 (alk. paper)
   1. Athletes–Mental health. 2. Sports–Psychological aspects, 3. Exercise–Psychological aspects. 4. Psychotherapy. 5. Exercise therapy. I. Hays, Kate F. II. Stern, E. Mark, 1929-   .
   [DNLM: 1. Athletic Injuries–rehabilitation. 2. Athletic Injuries–psychology. 3. Sports–psychology. 4. Exercise. 5. Movement. QT 261 I61 1998]
RC451.4.A83I56   1998
616.89′14′088796–dc21
DNLM/DLC
for Library of Congress   97-51665
                                                                        CIP

ISBN 13: 978-0-7890-0384-3 (pbk)

Integrating Exercise, Sports, Movement and Mind: Therapeutic Unity

CONTENTS

ABOUT THE EDITOR

Kate F. Hays, PhD, is a clinical and sport psychologist whose consulting practice, *The Performing Edge*, addresses the needs of athletes, performing artists, and business people. She has recently relocated to Toronto, following a 25-year practice in New Hampshire. She has lectured widely and written for professional and lay audiences on professional training in the practice of sport psychology. Dr. Hays is a Fellow of the American Psychological Association and a Certified Consultant, Association for the Advancement of Applied Sport Psychology.

ABOUT THE SERIES EDITOR

E. Mark Stern, EdD, ABPP, is Professor Emeritus in the Graduate Faculty of Arts and Sciences, Iona College, New Rochelle, New York. A Diplomate in Clinical Psychology of the American Board of Professional Psychology and a Fellow of the American Psychological Association, the American Psychological Society, and the Academy of Clinical Psychology, Dr. Stern has been President of the Divisions of Humanistic Psychology and Psychology of Religion, APA. He is in private practice of psychotherapy with offices at 215 East Eleventh Street, New York, NY 10003.

Preface

I treat the sports injured. No not the injured knee caps, nor the strained ankles. Rather much of my task is treating people who have clearly been injured by the "shortcomings" in their physical agility. For some, therapy has provided clear shifts in attitude, resulting in a more expansive physical hardiness.

Fred is a fine example. Up to the age of eight, he would shoot baskets in his backyard with his three older brothers. Looking back, Fred felt affection "the way a cute mascot probably feels." These warm beginnings gave way to confrontations with his own peers. In school and on the play fields he was pitted against boys his own size and age. And he fell short. Competition became more serious. Others had more ability. Fred was essentially excluded. Whether on the baseball diamond or across the volley ball net, Fred felt awkward. He was regularly belittled for his ineptitude and awkwardness.

Although Fred held his own grade-wise, he soon became reluctant to interact with his classmates. The school guidance counselor was unable to earn Fred's confidence. After a conference with the parents, Fred was referred to me. In a note to me, the school counselor commented that Fred was "forever excusing" for himself in inappropriate ways.

Fred hit it off with me. My not being linked to the school appeared to be a plus for our emerging relationship. From the first, Fred described himself as clumsy. Despite this negative derogation, I asked him to consider what he thought was possible for him. He asked me to help him with the question. I promised on condition that we both try to gain a perspective on all possibilities. I suggested that we'd have to be adventuresome. And that he probably never had had much of a chance to meet himself in the way we'd go about it. He smiled.

It took no time to achieve some common ground. I proposed that everyone has hidden potentialities. Looking for whatever was needed to

[Haworth co-indexing entry note]: "Preface." Stern, E. Mark. Co-published simultaneously in *The Psychotherapy Patient* (The Haworth Press, Inc.) Vol. 10, No. 3/4, 1998, pp. xi-xiii; and: *Integrating Exercise, Sports, Movement and Mind: Therapeutic Unity* (ed: Kate F. Hays) The Haworth Press, Inc., 1998, pp. xi-xiii. Single or multiple copies of this article are available for a fee from The Haworth Document Delivery Service [1-800-342-9678, 9:00 a.m. - 5:00 p.m. (EST). E-mail address: getinfo@haworth.com].

launch those desired capacities would take effort. I asked him to think about what could be blocking him in making the "moves" to make happen what he wanted to happen. Fred had always believed there were "crisis" differences between himself and his peers. He did indeed feel safer with older kids, more his brothers' ages. With them, he rarely felt taunted.

Fred could never "keep up" with boys his own age. Despite this "indelible curse," he felt master of "anything and everything in his own private world." Although he wouldn't or couldn't be specific, I asked him to cooperate in opening his "yet to be discovered worlds." Quite coincidentally, I was informed about an "Outward Bound"-type experience. It was to take place over an upcoming three-day weekend. It was to be guided by a young man with solid experience in helping kids overcome fears of the "wilderness." This particular expedition provided an excellent opportunity for physically awkward boys. The camping adventure was billed as challenging, and offering a facilitated group process before, during and after each day's journey. With his parents' blessings, Fred consented to go. I promised him that I would be available to talk to him the day after he returned.

The six other boys were slightly younger than Fred. The group was sparsely equipped. The idea was to learn the joys of hiking in order to arrive at a sense of survival in other challenging situations. Before taking off, the boys met as a group. They explored their apprehensions and were given assurances by the guide that he'd never be beyond sight and earshot of any of them. Fred's apprehensions were of another order. He feared not being sure-footed enough and being teased.

Fred did find himself lagging behind the others on the trail. Exclusion, no matter what the cause, did little to uplift his spirit. His discomfort intensified. Just as things appeared to be getting worse, Fred found himself joined by another boy. This one reliable friend-to-be "checked out" their position relative to the others. At first Fred was taken aback. But soon the new companion shared with Fred fears of his own, in particular of being singled out as a "slow poke." He joshed about how his feet didn't seem to coordinate properly. Fred, now in a position where he was able to give reassurance, suggested that they both take "swift" action. Encouraging each other, they gained on the others. Fred "amazed" himself with his own exuberance. Maintaining the pace did not come easy. But it *was* possible. Being with the group took on new meaning. Fred had experienced an unfamiliar potential. Flexibility replaced the rigidity he had learned throughout his life.

Back in therapy, Fred and I explored the way fear has of "freezing" people in place. I reminded him how free he felt shooting baskets with his older siblings. Yet something in him learned to believe that boys his own age were forbidding. I wanted to help Fred experience some new levels of sensory awareness. I asked him to make even more rigid the rigidity he felt in his physical bearing. Then I instructed him to let go of the tightness. Back and forth: tightness and ease; tension and freedom.

We began to explore the way bodily tension might have served him. The exercises of intensifying his disturbances allowed him to reflect on how even hurts interplay with personal utility. Ruling himself out had been one way of feeling "safe." If he had to endure kinesthetic defeat in order to achieve safety, then failure might have to be seen as somewhat adaptive. Fred was intrigued with the possibility that failing was an option that might sometimes be seen as freeing oneself from harm's way. He decided that he could also choose to risk a bit more as he had done on the hiking trails.

We focused on Fred's learning to recognize what his body was trying to tell him. I introduced some expansive imagery as one means of helping him regenerate his physical agility. This involved concentrating on some of the smallest movements he'd grown uncomfortably accustomed to. Eventually he came to accept that fears of failure might result in terrified contractions. The work of therapy enabled Fred to explore and experience an expanded repertoire of physical and social participation.

This assembly of research, practice and speculation is meant, among other things, for experienced psychotherapists to help more people like Fred. The samples of work and practice that Dr. Hays has assembled address themselves to modes of treating athletes, dancers and others who want to make more contact with their physical and emotional potentialities. The ever-changing roles of practicing psychotherapists are bound to interact with athletic coaches, teachers and practitioners of sports medicine. As with Fred, the redefinition of physical change comes about as does the enlargement of what is known of the psychology of the person. The discourses and interviews you are about to read are diverse, yet each one is meant to render its own means of helping individuals thrive both physically and emotionally.

E. Mark Stern
The Psychotherapy Patient *Series Editor*

Introduction

Kate F. Hays

The different prisms of exercise, sport, movement, and psychology interact to form a kaleidoscope design. Each element, multihued and multi-faceted in its own right, changes in tumbled juxtaposition to the others. Every revolution–whether the movement causes an individual element to change or produces new configurations–shifts patterns and connections. These permutations create endlessly fascinating challenges.

We do not have, in the English language, a name for this complex interaction–mindbody or bodymind. (Even that quintessentially words-strung-together language, German, can do no better than Leib-Seele-Einheit, or body-mind-unity.) "Psychosomatic" carries with it the implication of disease, the menacing and pejorative encroachment of a diseased mind on an innocent body. Because of its novelty, the term "somatopsychic," recently neologized by sport psychologist Wes Sime, allows us to pause briefly as we reflect on the effects of physical action on our thoughts and feelings.

Exercise psychology, the use of exercise to augment mental as well as physical health, is distinguished at times from sport psychology. The latter focuses more on competitive sport, and the mental aspects of the game, whether that be as specific as particular cognitive techniques or as broad as issues of motivation and team cohesion. Various movement therapies make use of the body's action to bypass verbal, left-brain, defensive knowing and reveal other experiential understandings.

Picture a kaleidoscope. Not the cheap black plastic tube that you rotate in order to change its patterns. Rather, a hand-constructed kaleidoscope, its wood grain burnished. Perhaps it is composed of multiple sections of glass bits. Your slightest movement, one way or the other, shifts the refracted images. Each sliver of colored glass is its own self while simultaneously

[Haworth co-indexing entry note]: "Introduction." Hays, Kate F. Co-published simultaneously in *The Psychotherapy Patient* (The Haworth Press, Inc.) Vol. 10, No. 3/4, 1998, pp. 1-3; and: *Integrating Exercise, Sports, Movement and Mind: Therapeutic Unity* (ed: Kate F. Hays) The Haworth Press, Inc., 1998, pp. 1-3. Single or multiple copies of this article are available for a fee from The Haworth Document Delivery Service [1-800-342-9678, 9:00 a.m. - 5:00 p.m. (EST). E-mail address: getinfo@haworth.com].

connecting and reconnecting with other shards in endless new patterns. Consider, now, the facets of these fields of inquiry, this multihued intersection of exercise, sport, body, movement, and mind.

Each article in this collection is designed to provide an interlocking element of the whole. Reading any one paper aids in understanding the next ones and reflects back on the meaning of previous ones. By mixing theory and application, abstraction and case study, these selections span the spectrum: gender, class, ethnicity, family systems, triangulation, coaching, multiple role relationships, TNT, anxiety, psychopathology, mirroring, injury, health, EMDR and beyond, consultation, developmental stages, flow, differentiation. Engagement is described around the following sports and activities: gymnastics, soccer, dressage (horseback riding), dance, skiing, running, walking, group activities, "child's play," archery, basketball, baseball, tennis, wrestling, football, and cycling.

Like the range of article topics and contents, the authors themselves were deliberately selected to reflect the many perspectives within this field. They bring to their articles a number of academic traditions, including in addition to clinical, counseling and social psychology, sport science, pastoral counseling, dance instruction, and occupational and physical therapy. Additionally, the voice of the performer shines through, whether as co-writer or permission-giving subject.

As "first keeper" of the kaleidoscope of these articles, I had the task of fixing some of the near connections. Organizing these articles into segments that speak directly to each other, I have perhaps arbitrarily located these connections at their points of similarity rather than contrast. The overall pattern moves from general frameworks to specific cases, although each article speaks to both theory and practice. In the first section, "Theoretical Frameworks," Stainback and La Marche apply family systems perspectives to youth sport; Heil, Wakefield, and Reed discuss injury rehabilitation via the metaphor "patient as athlete"; and Stern elaborates the movement-meaning interface via interviews with practitioners of dance therapy and Contact Improvisation. New light is just emerging on social issues in relation to sport and exercise. In the next section, "Gender, Ethnicity, and Class," Bacon, Fenby, and Lawrence make use of qualitative research to explore the experience of "flow" from within a gendered consciousness; Wildman provides a personal illustration of father-daughter sports interaction through the lens of relational theory; and Hall disentangles and reweaves the complexities of gender, class, and ethnicity in relation to exercise. The explosive interest in and development of sport psychology consultation over the past few decades has resulted in practitioners' need to understand and work within the coach/athlete/consultant triad. The authors of the next two papers, focused on sport psychology consultation, Van Raalte, and Gould and Damarjian, bring to their work a knowledge base of all angles of that triad. In the final set of papers, "Client Voices," detailed case histories refract the broader sweep indicated in earlier articles. Cogan picks up themes related to athletic retirement, consultation, and systems issues. Bauman and Carr examine injury recovery, visibility/notoriety, and cutting-edge treatment methods, and Petrie's client brings to the fore issues relating to ethnicity, injury recovery, and consultation.

As reader of these articles, you bring your own particular perspective to this kaleidoscope. Your lens of knowing colors your own reading. Further, the varied angles of these articles can provide an opportunity to reflect back on your everyday encounters with performance in multiple spheres. They can extend your knowledge; their references can, further, direct you toward additional learning. As true teachers, the authors of these articles lead us toward even further knowing.

For a time after I have been to an art museum, I use my eye in the same manner, observing the sights and textures of my surroundings as if through the lens I bring to viewing art. I note the Hopper-esque light on city buildings, the Mary Cassatt-like tenderness between parent and child, the Renaissance chiseling of a stranger's face, or a Turner-swirled sunset. As you, the reader, take in the kaleidoscope of these articles, I hope that you will experience ways in which the information in this volume infuses the ordinary ingredients of daily living.

For their eagle-eyed yet collegial comments on early drafts of these articles, I extend my grateful thanks to the following reviewers: Britton Brewer, Frances Flint, Sandra Foster, Diane Gill, Doreen Greenberg, Shane Murphy, Carole Oglesby, and Michael Sachs.

THEORETICAL FRAMEWORKS

Family Systems Issues
Affecting Athletic Performance in Youth

Robert D. Stainback
Judith A. La Marche

SUMMARY. Applying family systems constructs when working with
the developmental young athlete provides a comprehensive, interactive framework that integrates multiple issues into a unifying
theoretical model for understanding behavior and enhancing performance. This article describes basic family systems constructs, discusses the relevance to sport, and incorporates illustrative case
examples. The family "system" is defined broadly, referring to all
individuals who influence the athlete, including the spheres of fam-

---

Robert D. Stainback, PhD, is affiliated with the Veterans Administration Medical Center, Birmingham, AL.

Judith A. La Marche, PhD, is affiliated with the University of Alabama School
of Medicine, Birmingham, AL.

Correspondence should be addressed to: Robert D. Stainback, Birmingham
Veterans Administration Medical Center, 1717 11th Avenue South, Room 631,
Birmingham, AL 35205.

[Haworth co-indexing entry note]: "Family Systems Issues Affecting Athletic Performance in
Youth." Stainback, Robert D., and Judith A. La Marche. Co-published simultaneously in *The Psycho-
therapy Patient* (The Haworth Press, Inc.) Vol. 10, No. 3/4, 1998, pp. 5-20; and: *Integrating Exercise,
Sports, Movement and Mind: Therapeutic Unity* (ed: Kate F. Hays) The Haworth Press, Inc., 1998,
pp. 5-20. Single or multiple copies of this article are available for a fee from The Haworth Document
Delivery Service [1-800-342-9678, 9:00 a.m. - 5:00 p.m. (EST). E-mail address: getinfo@haworth.com].

ily (parents, siblings, and blended family members); sport (coaches, trainers, and team members); and school (teachers and social peers). The systems paradigm offers another perspective for the therapist to understand, evaluate, and treat the young athlete. *[Article copies available for a fee from The Haworth Document Delivery Service: 1-800-342-9678. E-mail address: getinfo@haworth.com]*

Dan Jansen, a favorite for the gold medal, fell barely 10 seconds into the 500-meter speed skating event at the 1988 Olympics in Calgary. A similar fate awaited him in the 1000-meter event where he also was among the favorites (Loehr, 1994). How could these unlikely events happen to a superbly trained, dedicated athlete who was apparently destined for stardom in Calgary? Earlier in the day of his first race, Dan's sister, Jane, had passed away. Coming from a closely-knit family, Dan was understandably shaken by his sister's death and apparently unable to fulfill his potential at the Olympics. However, these same strong family ties supported Dan through his future training and later successes, including an Olympic Gold Medal in the 1994 Games in Lillehammer.

Dan Jansen's story exemplifies the influences of an athlete's family of origin on athletic performance. In addition to the family of origin, there are numerous other individuals who may have an important influence on the young athlete. These significant individuals, along with the family of origin, comprise what has been referred to as a system. In youth sport (usually ages 5-21), this system may include a variety of persons, such as those from: the sport arena, e.g., coaches, trainers, health professionals, and other competitors; the school setting, e.g., teachers and peers; and the home, e.g., parents, siblings, and other significant family members (May & Brown, 1989). For purposes of this article, the term *family* refers to the family of origin and the term *system* connotes the entire network of individuals, both inside and outside of the family of origin, that may influence the athlete.

Therapists who work with performance enhancement in sport are well aware of the importance of emotional relationships for an athlete (Loehr, 1994). Children often learn about themselves and their world by patterns of behavior, communication of values, and personal relationships associated with organized sport. For better or worse, self-esteem is formulated and future behavior is shaped by this feedback (Danish, Petitpas, & Hale, 1990). Athletics, particularly youth sports, is believed to build character, stimulate hard work, and increase achievement motivation (Browne & Francis, 1993). However, excessive commitment to sport can have negative effects on the child, including: a narrowly focused identity which limits exploration of other skills; and an over-emphasis on winning which contributes to burnout, overuse injury, or use of feigned injury to avoid competitive pressure (Lidstone, Amundson, & Amundson, 1991; Petitpas & Danish, 1995).

The interdependence required in sport between the athlete, team participants, parents, teachers, coaches and others suggests that when professional assistance is indicated, a systemic approach to intervention may be effective (Hellstedt, 1995). The systems model may be particularly relevant to team consultation. Acknowledging that the interactions of system members may affect performance affords the therapist an opportunity to share observations, clarify patterns of communication and power, and identify issues needing resolution. Based in studies of group cohesion and structural systems, this theoretical framework offers a rationale for athletic performance–explaining why people do what they do (Zimmerman, Protinsky, & Zimmerman, 1994). That there is a system, or network of individuals, in all persons' lives that has a profound influence on their behavior is not a new idea. Systems theory suggests that a constellation of complex, interactive, and dynamic forces influences related individuals. Consultants have applied the systems model successfully to business and other organizations, but until recently, the relevance of the systems paradigm to sport has been overlooked (May & Brown, 1989; Zimmerman, Protinsky, & Zimmerman, 1994).

The remaining portions of this article provide a brief history of systems theory and a presentation of pertinent theoretical constructs with case examples to illustrate how systems issues affect sport performance. The identifying information of cases (seen by the first author) has been altered to protect confidentiality.

SYSTEMS ISSUES IN SPORT

Historical Overview of Systems Theory

The history of systems theory can be traced to pioneers such as Ackerman, Whitaker, and Bateson in the 1940s, followed by more contemporary theorists including Bowen, Satir, Jackson, Minuchin, and Haley. The system comprises a psychosocial unit, with focus on information processing, feedback mechanisms, and patterns of communication (Becvar & Becvar, 1988). Barker (1992) comprehensively reviews the literature on systems theory, and an excellent historical perspective is provided in a timeline of theoretical developments by Becvar and Becvar (1988, pp. 51-59).

A systems theoretical framework is unusual in that treatment modalities

may include any orientation, e.g., psychoanalytic, cognitive, behavioral, humanistic, gestalt, etc. (Becvar & Becvar, 1988). While cognitive behavioral orientations have been the mainstay of applied sport psychology, other approaches that have been applied to sport include hypnosis, neuro-linguistic programming, and reality and insight therapies. All of these approaches can be readily incorporated within a systems perspective (May & Brown, 1989).

Systems Theory and Sport

Natural tension occurs as a family unit must deal with a young athlete's developmental striving for mastery and autonomy. Summarizing developmental studies, Hellstedt (1995) provides a thorough review of stages and major tasks confronting the athlete's family. A playful early phase (ages 4-12) emphasizes fun and family involvement, traditionally associated with the father; an adolescent middle stage (ages 13-18) shifts the focus from the family to the coach for greater skill preparation and performance demand; and a later period (19-20s) launches the young athlete from childhood into independence and adulthood. In the first phase, while the focused structure of athletic activity lends harmony, an excessive sports emphasis distorts the balance of a young family. This can be seen in the "stage mother" and "star" phenomenon in many families. In adolescence, the power hierarchy of the family is altered, as boundaries are broadened to include coaches as well as teachers and peers. Here the adolescent may be challenging authority, a time of testing and turmoil. For the young adult, the athletic commitment may delay normal social maturation, extending financial and emotional dependence on the family unit. Clinical research regarding the perceptions of young athletes has revealed that emotional concomitants to competitive sport can be either positive or negative: verbal and nonverbal support by parents and siblings was regarded as beneficial by athletes; while worry, unrealistic expectations, and over involvement by family members were identified as detrimental influences (Hellstedt, 1995).

The effective therapist who works with young athletes takes a positive, active view of the family, identifying strengths, resources, and solutions for health and performance enhancement (Waters & Lawrence, 1993). Intervention is conducted *with* rather than *to*, acknowledging that the priorities, plans, and solutions are generated by the system, whose members are seen as capable and competent individuals. The therapist facilitates identification and understanding of system structure, roles, and repetitive behavioral and communication patterns (Zimmerman, Protinsky, & Zimmerman, 1994). Ongoing process evaluation consolidates learning and

provides the opportunity to experiment and to celebrate positive changes; successful engagement and mastery of challenges engenders feelings of courage, competence, and confidence (Hellstedt, 1995). With the focus broadened to a dynamic, interactive, multidimensional perspective, systems theory provides a uniquely comprehensive theoretical framework for working with athletes (Zimmerman & Protinsky, 1993).

THEORETICAL CONSTRUCTS IN SYSTEMS APPROACHES

A common systems lineage of research, theory, and applied development underlies current applications. The systems paradigm offers a comprehensive, integrative approach to youth sport intervention. The concepts presented in this article are those most relevant to the systems-sport interface.

Homeostasis

Most families are anxious to complain but reluctant to change. The family has developed patterns of communication and behavior which it will strive to maintain. This is an entirely understandable phenomenon from the systems viewpoint. When faced with stress (either positive or negative change) people naturally cling to stability for security. This desire to maintain the status quo is referred to as homeostasis (Watzlawick, Beavin, & Jackson, 1967). In systems theory, the presenting issues are seen as a clinical representation of the interplay between the family which strives for relative constancy, or homeostasis, and the ever-changing environment (Jackson, 1957; Raush, Greif, & Nugent, 1979). The first intervention issue is often that some authority must be relinquished to the therapist, thereby shifting the balance of power and threatening system homeostasis. This provides the therapist with an opportunity to discuss stressors internal as well as external to the system in a forthright manner, modeling trust and power sharing. These are key elements in learning to positively adapt to change.

Patterns of Communication

Both verbal and nonverbal expressions of system members function to maintain homeostasis (Watzlawick, Beavin, & Jackson, 1967). However, as conditions and events change, the family stability is challenged. This is particularly the case for young athletes who experience a plethora of

influences beyond family control. The child may feel distressed, caught between opposing expectations. Troubled families often convey messages in a confusing, contradictory, or subtly incongruent fashion. Bateson developed the concept of a "double-bind" to describe communication which carries an implicit conflict whereby any outcome will be painful, the situation has no escape, and the situation cannot be discussed (Barker, 1992). These circumstances become increasingly complex for the student athlete who strives to comply with contradictory messages from parents, coaches, teachers, siblings, and peers.

For example, 18-year-old Matt was a highly recruited, All-State tight end who could afford to go to college only if he received a scholarship. His father insisted that he excel at football, while his mother disparaged athletics and encouraged academics. Because both parents worked and he was the oldest of seven children, he had many responsibilities at home. His coaches expected him to devote 3 to 4 hours a day to team practice. Matt's performance became increasingly inconsistent. His parents complained that he was irresponsible, his teachers threatened academic probation, and his friends were annoyed with his distracted attention and angry outbursts. After several months of individual and family therapy, Matt and his family saw the impossible bind that conflicting expectations produced for him. Matt was encouraged to deal with the developmental issues of defining his own identity and goals, which then enabled him to sort out the conflicting messages. He began to feel greater control and self-esteem through making his own choices regarding lifestyle and activity. Matt had a good season, improved his grades, and enjoyed his social life. He enlisted greater assistance from his parents and his siblings, and began to focus on his class work. He accepted a football scholarship at the local junior college and decided to live at home.

Balance of Power: Hierarchy and Triangulation

The balance of power, an important concept in systems theory, refers to the location of power among and between family members (Minuchin & Fishman, 1982). In the case example of Matt, the balance of power and responsibility for the family was clarified as belonging to the parents. This acceptance led Matt's parents to work directly on resolving differing values. This improved their marital relationship and reduced Matt's tendency to feel caught in the crossfire of conflicting demands.

Hierarchy. Hierarchy refers to the generational boundaries of power. A typical adaptive hierarchy has a cohesive parental subsystem which is separated from that of the children. Healthy parents have greater power than their children and they cooperate as a couple with reciprocity and mutuality (Jacobs, 1991). Optimally, the adults operate in an increasingly egalitarian and flexible manner as the children mature. The positive development of adolescents has been found to be directly related to the cohesion, or emotional closeness, between family members (Gehring & Marti, 1993; Green, Harris, Forte, & Robinson, 1991). Two basic aspects of a healthy family, hierarchy and cohesion, are relatively stable characteristics throughout stress and change (Eckblad & Vandvik, 1992). Both a hierarchy reversal and a cross-generational coalition are considered sub-optimal family patterns (Gehring, 1990). The therapist can facilitate opportunities for success by assisting the system members in identifying maladaptive patterns, structuring tasks that are clear and attainable, and offering immediate and specific positive feedback that is age-appropriate.

A relatively common maladaptive pattern in youth sport is that of reversed generational boundaries, whereby the children or one child has greater power than the parents. For example, a family with an identified "star" displays a hierarchy reversal in which the child has greater power than a parent or sibling (ruling the roost). In many families where there is a star, there is often a sibling who compares unfavorably, and acts as a family scapegoat (Barker, 1992). This is sometimes referred to as the good child/bad child phenomenon.

Triangulation. The problems of a cross-generational coalition of the child with one parent against the other parent, or deflection of conflict between parents through focus on the child, are referred to as triangulation (Wood, 1993). According to Bowen (1978), an emotionally dependent parent, lacking in personal differentiation, creates anxiety and tension in the family. As alliances shift, conflict may occur between any two of the three role players. The isolated (triangulated) individual often strives to restore balance, feels caught in the middle, and/or may become the mutual enemy of the others. The couple may coalesce and stabilize around the child's problems, with the mother typically increasing attention and overprotectiveness while the father oscillates between providing criticism or support (Becvar & Becvar, 1988).

Minuchin (1974) describes relationship boundaries, both physical and emotional, along a continuum from disengagement to enmeshment. Dysfunctional families have difficulty finding and sustaining the appropriate balance. A parent-child dyad may form a cross-generational coalition (you and me against them). In youth sport, a maladaptive coalition may form if one parent aligns with a coach against the spouse. Often the coalition adheres to gender lines, as in the stereotypical example of the male athlete whose coach and father take a "pain equals weakness" attitude which conflicts with the "overprotective" mother who emphasizes health and safety. The athlete's alignment in these circumstances often reflects the balance of power in the system, i.e., the athlete will align with whomever he/she perceives as most powerful within the family.

Commenting on the triangulated interaction of coach/athlete/parent, Helstedt (1987) observed that coaches are often critical of interfering parents, but are reluctant to deal directly with them. In order to decrease triangulation, the coach can: (a) provide clear expectations based on explicit values and coaching philosophy; (b) engage in interactive communication regarding nutritional programs, training schedules, academic criteria, and sleep requirements; (c) encourage realistic goal setting and give honest feedback regarding the athlete's skill development; (d) inform and educate about the sport, the positions, and the strategies appropriate for that developmental age; and (e) have a procedure for dealing with individual problems (Helstedt, 1987).

The following case examples are intended to illustrate systems issues as they apply to youth sport. For each case example, the presenting problems will be described briefly, followed by a discussion of systems factors playing influential roles in the therapeutic change process.

CASE EXAMPLES

Kelly, a Gymnast

Kelly, a 12-year-old gymnast, had been involved in the sport since age 6. Although she previously enjoyed her participation, over the past year she had been showing signs of stress (e.g., not wanting to attend practice, anxiety about competitions, etc.). The coach referred her and her parents to the therapist due to her "obvious signs of discomfort while attending practices and competitions."

Kelly arrived at the initial evaluation session with her parents and 14-year-old sister, Anna. Her father initially was reluctant to participate in a family intervention, but came grudgingly at the insistence of his wife. Kelly presented as a rather awkward, reserved young girl who appeared larger both in height and weight than the average 12-year-old. In contrast, Anna and their mother both appeared petite, feminine, and self-confident. Anna, also a gymnast, stated that she enjoyed her competitive experiences. Her mother stated that, as a matter of fact, Anna was an honor student while consistently leading her team in state meets for the past 5 years.

Kelly's mother indicated that her younger daughter had shown diminishing interest in gymnastics over the last year. She expressed concern because she felt that gymnastics provided an excellent way for Kelly to get exercise and have fun, as well as meet and enjoy a variety of other children. Her mother mused that the girls did not have much in common outside of gymnastics, noting Kelly's academic difficulty and social awkwardness. Kelly started competing at the same age as her sister, but never garnered the same accolades and did not seem to share her sister's fervor for competition. Her mother believed Kelly's decreased interest in gymnastics was related to some negative experiences with competition. Kelly's mother did not feel that either the gymnastics coach or her husband had negatively influenced Kelly with regard to gymnastics. They all tried to treat Kelly in the same way they treated Anna, she commented. The family had centered their life around the gymnastics practices and meets for the past 9 years. Both parents summarized their thoughts in the first session by stating that they wanted what was best for Kelly and supported her regardless of her participation in gymnastics.

Kelly had some difficulty clearly expressing her feelings. She acknowledged that she always was nervous before competing, which made the experience unpleasant. According to Kelly, the best part of gymnastics was being around her friends. She would just as soon not compete, but, she stated in a tremulous voice, it seemed clear to her that if she did not compete, she would not measure up to her sister and would not be accepted by her friends in the gymnastics club. She reasoned that Anna would be relieved if she quit because she probably was an embarrassment to her sister. When asked if she talked with anyone else about her feelings, she indicated that she was reluctant to tell her parents and coach because she was afraid that they would be disappointed in her. She could not identify specifically what her parents and coach were doing or saying to lead her to feel this way. When asked if she had similar feelings with regard to her experiences at school, Kelly indicated that she also had difficulty taking tests because she felt she was being compared to her classmates by the teacher. She stated that this feeling was uncomfortable because "I just don't feel that I measure up." Reports from Kelly's school teachers indicated that her performance in school had declined in the last 6 months.

Case Analysis

This case example depicts: (a) how Kelly's difficulty in adjusting to competition challenged the family homeostasis; (b) how patterns of ineffective communication led to misunderstandings between Kelly and her family; and (c) how the unbalanced family power created an experience of isolation for Kelly. The system dynamics had negative effects on her self-esteem and social development. When competition was introduced at age 10, her failure relative to her "star" sister made her sport participation unpleasant. She clearly felt that she would disappoint adults who were important to her (mother, father, and coach) if she were to drop out of competitive gymnastics. She also apparently felt this bind with regard to her social status, thinking that if she discontinued, she would lose the relationships that sustained her. She recognized with bitter insight that coaches and teachers compared her to her sister and were disappointed in the contrast. With this self-appraisal, she lacked the confidence to engage in normal social activities even when her classmates invited her to join them.

The job for the therapist in this case was to help Kelly and her family identify the factors contributing to her dilemma. Kelly's parents had devoted the previous 9 years of their 15-year marriage to a life revolving around gymnastics competition. The marital couple had been using gymnastics to bridge gaps in their own relationship. Kelly's mother had left her promising career in marketing to devote herself to the children. Kelly's father felt the full responsibility for the family's financial welfare, and, in turn, devoted himself to his position at the bank. As their lives drifted apart, they shared little of the joy and affection which had characterized their early marriage. However, they reveled in the pleasure and pride of watching Anna's success. If only Kelly were more like her sister. . . .

What place was left for Kelly? Kelly's self-worth had been defined in terms of her ability to fit the family pattern. In treating her "just the same as her sister," they actually failed to look for and develop those talents which were uniquely Kelly's. Despite their statement of unconditional support for Kelly, not participating in gymnastics would leave Kelly alone in the afternoons and on weekends, both literally and emotionally. The family unit had developed a hierarchy reversal focused on Anna, leaving Kelly feeling like a dim bulb compared to their bright star.

What effect would change in Kelly's athletic activity have on the marital couple? On Anna? On Kelly? At first, it was hard for Anna and her parents to appreciate the pain in Kelly's dilemma. They knew that they loved her deeply. Yet their patterns of communication and behavior created the dilemma. Kelly had grown up understanding that the path to her parents' affection was via successful gymnastics competition. But Kelly was not Anna, and did not have the same physical talent or psychological drive as her sister. Kelly had a wonderful imagination and was artistically creative, but received little time, attention, or guidance for these talents. The reality of gymnastics competition demanded driving the girls to practices and meets, and that consumed every afternoon and weekend. Time or energy was not allocated to listen to Kelly's stories or glance at her sketches. Kelly wanted to establish her own identity, but feared that she would prove a failure to her parents and coach. If she quit gymnastics, she risked the loss of her common bond with her sister and the loss of team friendships.

Exploring family and subsystem balances of power, hierarchies, and interaction patterns is referred to as structural analysis (Barker, 1982). In this case, structural analysis revealed that the family unit was unbalanced, with parental power subjugated by the focus on Anna's gymnastics. Kelly felt that she was in a no-win situation. The marital relationship needed re-alignment with clearer generational boundaries; the siblings needed more individualized time and attention. Facilitated discussion helped Kelly identify her circumstances and gave credence to her feelings. In turn, this lessened her sense of confusion and isolation. Kelly and her family recognized that very little communication of each family member's needs, wants, or feelings took place. Gymnastics was always the topic of conversation and the focus of family activity. Through consultation, Kelly identified her own needs and wants, including the desire to teach gymnastics to preschoolers at the local YMCA on Saturdays and to take art lessons after school. Kelly had been afraid to approach her coach about quitting—nobody likes a quitter! To her surprise, the coach was supportive of her, and commented that she would be an excellent teacher. At school, her teacher and classmates noticed her new enthusiasm. Kelly's parents still enjoyed watching Anna's meets, but no longer expected Kelly to attend every competition. Anna joined a car pool so that her parents could now drive to practice for one week each month rather than every day after school. They were then available to arrange a car pool for Kelly's art classes. Interestingly, as therapy progressed, Kelly's parents became aware that other interests of their own had been neglected. They began to take more adult time, including having "a date" for dinner together on Saturday nights. Kelly's mother now had time to spend in the church and community activities that had been so important to her before she had devoted herself to gymnastics. Kelly's father found that he was feeling better. He now had more time to exercise after work, since he was not always picking up the girls. At first, Anna resisted the changes adamantly, but she later appreciated that she was afforded more independence through the process. Although she enjoyed the benefits of gymnastics, including the physical fitness, closeness with team members, affection for the coach, and positive self-esteem from successful competition, Anna sometimes had felt a heavy burden from the high expectations of her parents. She also found that she enjoyed being with her friends without her mother being there every day.

The patterns of communication now allowed family members to express their own desires and talents. Verbal exchanges led to behavioral experimentation. The therapist's intervention allowed an opportunity to realign the parental executive subsystem, re-establish the generational boundaries, and facilitate the individual differentiation of each child, particularly for Kelly. The family learned skills which they could use in times of future stress. Undoubtedly, there will be more challenges as the girls mature. Therefore, the marital couple's developing, cohesive parenting style (more adaptive hierarchy) will be valuable in meeting the future needs of the family.

Michael, a Soccer Player

At age 17, Michael was relatively small, but quite fast, with quick reactions. Given the accuracy of his kicking, these talents had made him an exceptional soccer forward. Following a serious injury to his leg, his mother commented that Michael "was not himself." After several months of diligent rehabilitative work, Michael was told by the rehabilitation medicine staff that his leg was as strong as ever. However, Michael's play was not returning to its previous level and he was showing attitude and behavior changes that worried his mother.

Michael and his mother came for the first session with the therapist. He was hesitant to talk during the first session and had difficulty maintaining eye contact. With reluctance, Michael admitted that he was having difficulty sleeping and had little appetite since preseason practice for soccer started several weeks ago. As this was the fall of his senior year, he was convinced that he needed to exceed his previous accomplishments in order to receive the college scholarship he so wanted. He felt that his high school coach, with whom he had a close relationship, depended on him to lead the team to the division championship. He also indicated that he felt pressure from his teammates to assume the same scoring role he had the previous year when he led the team and league in goals and assists. His team had finished second in the state last season. Although he hoped that he would be able to meet these expectations, Michael explained that he wasn't at all sure about himself and his skills since his injury. He also expressed fears about re-injuring himself and therefore disappointing himself, his teammates, and his coach.

Michael's mother disclosed that she had been divorced since her son was 3 years old, and that he had little contact with his father who lived in another state. Although she had established a successful career as a lawyer,

Michael was her only child and her "whole life." Consequently, she was very concerned about the seriousness of his injury and feared that he was returning to competitive sport too early. She indicated that although she would love it if he got a soccer scholarship, it was not worth risking his health. "All I want is for my son to be happy, enjoy his senior year in high school, and then see how things turn out for college."

In subsequent sessions, Michael continued to discuss his concerns about letting his teammates and coach down if he were unable to regain his previous performance levels. He also indicated that, as the start of the season was drawing closer, he was having increased apprehensions about whether his leg would hold up during a game. He further noted feeling some anxiety about his school work and his relationship with his girlfriend because all of his attention had been focused on soccer during the last month. He hoped that, after the season started, things would settle down and he would feel better about himself and his situation.

Sessions with Michael's mother proved interesting and apparently therapeutic for both Michael and his mother. She became aware that her general tendency was to make Michael the primary focus of her emotional life, that she harbored some resentment about his impending maturity and independence, and that she was communicating/behaving in an inconsistent fashion. For example, she said she hoped for a soccer scholarship, but really had misgivings about him leaving home. She indicated that she was anxious about how she would adjust when Michael graduated from high school and left for college. Understanding that this was a step she wanted him to take, she was supportive of him developing independence, but nonetheless was reluctant to see the time draw so close. With similar ambivalence, she acknowledged that, while she was proud of his accomplishments, she feared for his safety.

Case Analysis

In Michael's case, a serious injury affected the system homeostasis. Resultant increases in both external (coach and teammates) and internal (Michael) pressures led to an unbalanced, triangulated system. His injury, along with the prolonged period of recovery and requisite time away from competition, apparently had caused Michael to have concerns about his ability to reestablish himself as the team's emotional and scoring leader. Although perhaps not directly communicated by his coach and teammates, Michael felt that he must return to previous levels of performance in order to maintain the team's former success (i.e., preserve the homeostasis of the system). Given his performance insecurity, he was in a tenuous emotional situation that might actually make him more vulnerable to re-injury (Andersen & Williams, 1988; Rose & Jevne, 1993). For instance, he might attempt to push himself too hard to assume the leadership responsibilities he perceived that his coach was expecting of him and therefore not pay attention to bodily cues that warn of injury risk (e.g., soreness, fatigue, etc.).

The boundaries between mother, coach, and son were not well-defined, particularly following Michael's injury. The disparity between his mother's and the coach's expectations widened. Michael found himself in the position of choosing between playing harder (the coach) or playing less (his mother), presenting an impossible bind. These concerns added to his anxiety, disrupting his performance. Michael and his coach focused on his athletic performance. Although he displayed physical signs of emotional distress (sleep and eating disturbance, poor school performance, and difficulty in social relationships), neither he nor his coach recognized these as stress symptoms. The alliance between Michael and his coach left his mother feeling isolated. In response to a sense of powerlessness, she increased her apprehension and protectiveness.

Given the dynamics involved in Michael's situation, therapy sessions were spent not only with Michael individually, but also with Michael and his mother, coach, and a selected few of his teammates. Individual sessions with Michael focused on clarifying his own concerns and expectations about returning to competition. With these considerations better identified, joint sessions with other members of the system focused on communicating these concerns and soliciting open discussions about them. The goal was to identify the accuracy of Michael's concerns regarding the expectations of others within the system and to begin resolving discrepancies between expectations. These sessions proved to be beneficial to all parties. Michael found that while his coach and teammates had high expectations for the team this season, they realized that he needed time to re-establish himself. Several teammates felt that scoring responsibilities and leadership could be successfully distributed among team members, thereby sharing the pressure. The coach expressed similar thoughts, but also indicated that everyone was anxious to see Michael back on the field.

Interventions used in this case were geared toward establishing clearer relationship boundaries. Michael was able to communicate his concerns more openly which led to greater understanding by his mother, coach, and teammates. He was able to return to competition at a pace and expectation level that allowed him to resume his role within the team gradually. Teammates were able to adjust accordingly and contribute more to the scoring and leadership responsibilities. Michael's mother began to accept the impending departure of her son to college and was able to refocus her attention to the positive aspects of this developmental step for both her son and herself.

CONCLUSION

The family systems model offers an integrated theoretical approach to understanding behavioral dynamics commonly observed in the sport arena. Perhaps not in any other therapeutic situation are the dynamics of systems so pronounced as in youth sport. A visit to a neighborhood field or gymnasium to study the interactions of youngsters, parents, and coaches will illustrate the point. The face validity of systems theory constructs becomes readily apparent.

Although further research is needed, a systemic approach appears conducive to youth sport intervention, providing a comprehensive framework for understanding issues affecting athletic performance and theoretical schemata from which appropriate interventions can be applied throughout the athlete's development (Hellstedt, 1995). Practitioners are encouraged to consider using a systems perspective to understand, evaluate, and treat the young athlete.

REFERENCES

Andersen, M. B. & Williams, J. M. (1988). A model of stress and athletic injury: Prediction and prevention. *Journal of Sport & Exercise Psychology, 10,* 294-306.

Barker, P. (1992). *Basic family therapy* (3rd ed.). New York: Oxford University Press.

Becvar, D. S. & Becvar, R. J. (1988). *Family therapy: A systemic integration.* Boston: Allyn & Bacon, Inc.

Bowen, M. (1978). *Family therapy in clinical practice.* New York: Jason Aronson.

Browne, B. A., & Francis, S. K. (1993). Participants in school-sponsored and independent sports: Perceptions of self and family. *Adolescence, 28, 383-391.*

Danish, S. J., Petitpas, A. J., & Hale, B. D. (1990). Sport as a context for developing competence. In T. Gullotta, G. Adams, & R. Montemayor (Eds.), *Developing social competence in adolescence: Vol. 3* (pp. 169-194). Newberry Park, CA: Sage.

Eckblad, G. & Vandvik, I. H. (1992). A computerized scoring procedure for the Kvebaek family sculpture technique applied to families of children with rheumatic diseases. *Family Process, 31, 85-98.*

Gehring, T. M. (1990). The Family System Test (FAST). In B. F. Perlmutter, M. A. Straus & J. Touliatos (Eds). *Handbook of family measurement techniques* (pp. 113-114). Newbury Park, CA: Sage Publication.

Gehring, T. M. & Marti, D. (1993). The Family System Test: Differences in perception of family structures between nonclinical and clinical children. *Journal of Child Psychology, Psychiatry, & Allied Disciplines, 34,* 363-377.

Green, R. G., Harris, R. N., Forte, J. A., & Robinson, M. (1991). Evaluating

FACES III Systems and the circumplex model: 2,440 families. *Family Process, 30,* 55-73.

Hellstedt, J. C. (1987). The coach/parent/athlete relationship. *The Sport Psychologist, 1,* 151-160.

Hellstedt, J. C. (1995). Invisible players: A family systems model. In S. M. Murphy (Ed.), *Sport psychology interventions* (pp. 117-147). Champaign, IL: Human Kinetics.

Jackson, D. D. (1957). The question of family homeostasis. *Psychiatric Quarterly Supplement, 1(1),* 79-90.

Jacobs, E. H. (1991). Self psychology and family therapy. *American Journal of Psychotherapy, 45,* 483-498.

Lidstone, J. E., Amundson, M. L., & Amundson, L. H. (1991). Depression and chronic fatigue in the high school student and athlete. *Primary Care, 18,* 283-296.

Loehr, J. E. (1994). *The new toughness training for sport.* New York, NY: Dutton.

May, J. R. & Brown, L. (1989). Delivery of psychological services to the U.S. Alpine Ski Team prior to and during the Olympics in Calgary. *The Sport Psychologist, 3,* 320-329.

Minuchin, S. (1974). *Families and family therapy.* Cambridge, MA: Harvard University Press.

Minuchin, S., & Fishman, H. C. (1982). *Techniques of family therapy.* Cambridge, MA: Harvard University Press.

Petitpas, A. & Danish, S. J. (1995). Caring for injured athletes. In S. M. Murphy (Ed.), *Sport psychology interventions* (pp. 255-283). Champaign, IL: Human Kinetics.

Raush, H.L., Greif, A.C., & Nugent, J. (1979). Communication in couples and families. In W.R. Burr, R. Kill, F. I. Nye, & I. L. Reiss (Eds.), *Contemporary theories about the family: Vol. 1, Research-based theories* (pp. 468-489). New York: The Free Press.

Rose, J. & Jevne, R. F. J. (1993). Psychosocial processes associated with athletic injuries. *The Sport Psychologist, 7,* 309-328.

Waters, D. B. & Lawrence, E. C. (1993). *Competence, courage, and change: An approach to family therapy* New York: W. W. Norton & Company.

Watzlawick, P., Beavin, J. H., & Jackson, D. D. (1967). *Pragmatics of human communication: A study of interactional patterns, pathologies, and paradoxes.* New York: W. W. Norton & Company.

Wood, B. L. (1993). Beyond the "psychosomatic family": A biobehavioral family model of pediatric illness. *Family Process, 32,* 261-278.

Zimmerman, T. S. & Protinsky, H. (1993). Uncommon sports psychology: consultation using family therapy theory and techniques. *The American Journal of Family Therapy, 21,* 161-174.

Zimmerman, T. S., Protinsky, H. O., & Zimmerman, C. S. (1994). Family systems consultation with an athletic team: A case study of themes. *Journal of Applied Sport Psychology, 6,* 101-115.

Patient as Athlete:
A Metaphor for Injury Rehabilitation

John Heil
Carla Wakefield
Cherrine Reed

SUMMARY. Conceptualizing injury rehabilitation as an athletic challenge illuminates the process of rehabilitation for patient and psychologist. This approach synthesizes behavioral medicine and sport psychology to create a model that identifies psychological roles for all members of the treatment team and empowers patients by a proactive approach to education and skill-building. The development of the patient-athlete mind-set is a common focus across all interventions. The patient-athlete mind-set encompasses: personal responsibility, a strong goal orientation, readiness to pursue physical training with intensity and precision, and a willingness to move one's physical and mental skills to a higher level of performance. A case example of a recreational athlete suffering chronic pain illustrates the patient-athlete metaphor. *[Article copies available for a fee from The Haworth Document Delivery Service: 1-800-342-9678. E-mail address: getinfo@haworth.com]*

Injury rehabilitation challenges mind and body. Traditionally, recovery from injury has been a passive sit-and-wait endeavor (Berryman, 1995). In

John Heil, DA, is affiliated with the Lewis-Gale Clinic and the Lewis-Gale Hospital Pain Management Center.

Carla Wakefield, OTR, is affiliated with the Lewis-Gale Hospital Pain Management Center.

Cherrine Reed, PT, is affiliated with the Lewis-Gale Hospital Pain Management Center.

[Haworth co-indexing entry note]: "Patient as Athlete: A Metaphor for Injury Rehabilitation." Heil, John, Carla Wakefield, and Cherrine Reed. Co-published simultaneously in *The Psychotherapy Patient* (The Haworth Press, Inc.) Vol. 10, No. 3/4, 1998, pp. 21-39; and: *Integrating Exercise, Sports, Movement and Mind: Therapeutic Unity* (ed: Kate F. Hays) The Haworth Press, Inc., 1998, pp. 21-39. Single or multiple copies of this article are available for a fee from The Haworth Document Delivery Service [1-800-342-9678, 9:00 a.m. - 5:00 p.m. (EST). E-mail address: getinfo@haworth.com].

stark contrast, sports medicine prescribes active vigorous rehabilitation and champions the metaphor "every patient an athlete." A growing body of evidence suggests that the patient's thoughts and behaviors affect the speed and thoroughness of recovery and the psychological impact of injury (e.g., Ievleva & Orlick, 1991). The goal of this paper is to present a psychology of injury rehabilitation that is based on the metaphor of "patient as athlete." A perspective on treatment is provided that extends the proactive sports medicine philosophy into the mental realm by drawing on the principles and practices of sport psychology. Thus, guiding the patient in thinking and acting like an athlete becomes a central goal of rehabilitation.

SPORT PSYCHOLOGY, CHRONIC PAIN, AND ATHLETICISM

This section begins with a brief overview of two distinct topics, sport psychology and chronic pain, that will be integrated through the remainder of the paper. It also describes a continuum of athleticism and lays initial groundwork for developing related intervention strategies.

The major thrust of sport psychology, as it has developed over the last 25 years, involves training the athlete in mental skills to enhance performance within the stress of competitive environments (Browne & Mahoney, 1984; Druckman & Bjork, 1991). It is based on a pragmatic educational model which emphasizes the development of skills through psychologist-directed training and athlete-directed practice. Sport psychology focuses on motivation, goal setting, communication skills, group cohesion, and adaptations of traditional cognitive behavioral therapies, typically dubbed "mental training" (Henschen & Straub, 1995; Van Raalte & Brewer, 1996; Weinberg & Gould, 1995). While these methods are the standard fare of much psychological practice, they are distinctive in the way they have been adapted to address the individual needs of athletes and the competitive environments in which they train and compete (Browne & Mahoney, 1984). As sport psychology has matured, its practices and principles have been applied to increasingly diverse groups with the goal of improving performance. This includes business executives and performing artists as well as military, police, and public safety personnel (Orlick, 1990). Due to the ubiquitous nature of sport injury, practices that incorporate performance-enhancement principles have been developed to guide the rehabilitation of athletes. Our work extends this psychology of sport injury to general medical rehabilitation.

Chronic pain is a formidable but relatively common health care problem that is both a source of widespread unabated suffering and a tremendous financial burden to society at large. By current estimates, the cost of chronic low back pain in the United States will exceed $100 billion dollars by the year 2000 (Williams, 1995). Clinically, chronic pain is an enigma. It is widely misunderstood and often ineffectively treated, with the result that pain and its sequelae may be exacerbated rather than ameliorated (Bonica, 1991). Chronic pain patients are widely recognized as a treatment-resistant group and one clearly in need of highly specialized and incisively individualized treatment. In this population, the practitioner finds the universe of problems that may be encountered in injury rehabilitation, including: multiple persistent medical problems; psychological sequelae such as depression and anxiety; behavior problems (e.g., poor compliance, fear of reinjury); personality conflicts with treatment providers; and suspicion of malingering. Hence, chronic pain treatment requires a broad range of problem-solving strategies that integrate psychological and medical interventions. This is illustrated in the case example that appears later. Chronic pain is the segment of the injury rehabilitation population where psychological treatment is most widely accepted and most extensively applied and where the psychologist is generally recognized as a key team player. It is our impression that thinking and acting like an athlete embodies a set of attitudes and behaviors which can open the door to recovery in otherwise unsuccessful rehabilitation.

We suggest that the patient-athlete metaphor applies to all injured patients although the specifics of application differ. There is a continuum of athletic engagement from non-athlete to recreational athlete to elite athlete. As a general rule, to the extent that patients are athletes, their skills need to be *transferred* to the rehabilitation setting–and to the extent they are non-athletes, athletic skills need to be *trained*. Recreational athletes represent a substantial segment of the injury rehabilitation population, in contrast to elite athletes, who are relatively few in number. Recreational athletes may be more readily receptive to the patient-athlete metaphor than non-athletes. Hence, they are the ideal target group for the practitioner who wants to develop this treatment approach.

While this paper focuses on the recreational athlete, for the sake of thoroughness, a brief discussion of injury management among elite athletes and non-athletes follows. For the elite athlete, severe injury can be a bewildering and emotionally disrupting experience. The profound change in lifestyle that follows can threaten self-image and self-worth. The pressure to get well in a hurry can be tremendous. Work with the elite athlete focuses on the transfer of sport skills by reframing injury rehabilitation: it becomes an athletic challenge that has shifted from the playing field or arena to the rehabilitation center. This draws on the athlete's strengths, including mental discipline, goal setting, pain tolerance, and a strong proclivity for the physical training that is the basis of rehabilitation. With relative minor injury, the idea of transfer of skills is typically grasped quite readily. However, the more severe the injury, the more difficult it is for the elite athlete to understand the role of athleticism in rehabilitation. Sometimes this understanding can be built gradually; other times it may suddenly crystallize as a powerful insight. Fred was a collegiate conference leading hurdler with Olympic aspirations who suffered a disabling injury. Alter a protracted struggle to reorient to his new life situation, one day Fred said "I know what to do, I approach every day like a workout." He then explained the need for focused attention and emotional intensity to meet the rigor of the physical demands of day to day activity with a physical disability. Then he added, "In my mind, I'm still an athlete."

The non-athlete faced with a demanding course of rehabilitation can descend to the state of a traveler lost in the wilderness, wandering aimlessly in the hope of being rescued. What is needed is a plan that will direct the traveler through unfamiliar terrain and empower him or her as navigator of this journey. The treatment providers must train the patient step by step, day by day, in the essential skills of rehabilitation and in the concepts upon which these skills are based. The patient-athlete metaphor illuminates the principles of fitness and conditioning that rehabilitation and sport share in common, thus enabling patients to be active agents in their own care. In contrast to recreational or elite athletes, the practitioner should expect (among non-athletes) a relatively slow curve of physical functional improvement and conceptual understanding.

THE PATIENT-ATHLETE METAPHOR

The language of sport in the popular media abounds with reference to teamwork, fair play, making the big play, the thrill of victory, and so on. Considering the numbers involved in sport–directly through participation and indirectly through spectatorship–and the level of passion that accompanies this involvement, sport is clearly a formidable societal influence. As such, the concept of the "athlete" already exists as a metaphor deeply ingrained in the collective unconscious of Western society.

The athlete metaphor is both familiar and intrinsically appealing, one that can function both superficially and at conceptually rich levels. Superficially, an association with athleticism casts rehabilitation in a positive and upbeat light. Rehabilitation is thus defined as the challenge to body and mind that it truly is, by reference to the work ethic of athleticism: personal dedication, goal orientation, challenging practice regimens, pain tolerance, and striving to move to a higher level of performance. This comparison helps normalize the sometimes bewildering struggle in which patients find themselves embroiled. It legitimizes their suffering. When patients are referred by rehabilitation providers to psychologists, the athlete analogy assuages their concern that such a referral implies that they are "crazy" or that "the pain is all in their head." As the patient-athlete (like the athlete) works to build strength and endurance, flexibility and range of motion, the stage is set for teaching fundamental training concepts and cultivating the athlete mind set.

By the time most patients are diagnosed with chronic pain, they have tried and failed routine rehabilitation. This gives rise to a "sick role" that becomes increasingly entrenched with the chronicity of the pain (Fordyce, 1976). The patient is typically reluctant–sometimes doubting the efficacy of treatment or experiencing an outright fear of reinjury. In essence, the patient must abandon the attitude of passivity and helplessness that chronic pain engenders and find a new way to think about rehabilitation. A shift in perspective from "patient" to "patient-athlete" can foster a sense of independence and self-efficacy, provide a conceptual framework to guide rehabilitation, and move the individual to a higher level of performance.

THE PATIENT-ATHLETE IN ACTION

The patient-athlete is the key player in the game of rehabilitation. To regain health and function, the patient-athlete must be active, yet activity is a double-edged sword. When underdone, rehabilitation may plateau seemingly endlessly; and when overdone, may lead to a habitual cycle of injury exacerbation and emotional distress. When done with precision, rehabilitation proceeds on course. The treatment team guides the patient-athlete in the development of special knowledge and skills with an approach that begins as rehabilitation and segues into personal training. In the process, responsibility for directing treatment gradually shifts from the treatment team to the patient. There are four key elements of athleticism in rehabilitation: therapeutic exercise, aerobic exercise, resumption of lost recreational activity, and the development of the athlete mind-set.

Therapeutic Exercise

Therapeutic exercise is the cornerstone of injury rehabilitation. It is designed to restore lost strength, flexibility, and endurance. It also incorporates recommendations regarding "proper technique" (i.e., body mechanics, joint protection, etc.). Therapeutic regimens gradually progress in duration, frequency, and intensity. These fundamental skills serve as building blocks for the resumption of work, recreation, and other activities of daily living. Work hardening techniques bridge the gap between therapeutic exercise and work (or sport) by simulating specific work (or sport) activities in a carefully supervised environment. This facilitates skill development and independent function.

Therapeutic exercise regimens create an approach-avoidance conflict for the patient-athlete who desires to quickly regain lost function but fears reinjury, pain, and failure. Effective physical therapy and occupational therapy focus on realistic goals, positive expectations, and careful pacing of effort (Dole, Cracker, Muleteer, & Doleys, 1986; Fordyce et al., 1981). This cultivates self-efficacy and opens the door to a successful outcome as the patient-athlete carries these principles from therapy into work, sport, and other activities of daily living.

Aerobic Activity

Aerobic activity involves sustained increase in large muscle and cardiopulmonary activity. It yields a broad range of beneficial effects including total body fitness, improved sleep, weight loss, and pain relief via neurochemical production. Aerobic conditioning is an increasingly commonplace component of sport injury rehabilitation. It enables the athlete to maintain fitness and minimizes the feeling of loss that comes with relative inactivity (Steadman, 1982). Its use is critical because of the deconditioning (this rehabilitation term describes loss of fitness due to inactivity) commonly found in chronic pain patients. Gains in muscular endurance provide a foundation for work hardening and resumption of lost recreational activities. The mood enhancing effects help alleviate the depression and anxiety frequently linked to severe injury (Bozoian, Rejeski, & McCauley, 1994; Long & Van Stravel, 1995; Nicoloff & Schwenk, 1995). Successful engagement in aerobic activity challenges the "sick role" that is commonly seen in chronic pain. Because injury and pain create inherent limitations, patient-athletes may begin their aerobic type activity (for example, walking, cycling) at subaerobic levels. Intensity can be gradually increased to reach true aerobic activity.

Resumption of Lost Recreational Activity

The importance of sport activity to the recreational athlete is often undervalued and hence neglected by treatment providers. Work, family, and other responsibilities allow little time for other activities. Thus, those activities in which people *are* able to engage take on added significance, and as such their loss is sorely felt. The resumption of recreational activities is mood enhancing and helps to further challenge the "sick role" and sense of disability that characterizes the chronic pain patient.

When recreational activities can no longer be done in their customary fashion, they may be abandoned by the chronic pain patient. Resumption of activity begins with letting go of an "all or none" attitude towards recreation and with being willing to find satisfaction in some elements of the original activity. Consider the avid fly fisherman who relished wading remote and rugged streams searching for the elusive "big one." Resumption of activity could begin with fishing from the banks with the patient-athlete alternating between sitting and standing. Eventually, the patient-athlete can enter the stream in quiet water with a smooth bottom and gradually increase the time in the stream. As able, the patient-athlete may venture into the more challenging areas of the stream, taking periodic rest breaks as needed. No first step is too small. Those who are most severely limited may begin with a visit to the river to simply sit peacefully for a while. This can help foster a rediscovery of the pleasure of being in a natural setting–and help open the door to the progressive approach to resumption of recreation that has been described.

At times, recreational activity can function as the leading edge in the recovery process. The level of personal investment and skill of the committed recreational athlete fosters a resourcefulness not found in other activities. As such, recreation may serve as a vehicle for problem solving where progress has otherwise plateaued or stagnated.

Athlete Mind-Set

The patient-athlete metaphor developed throughout this paper has the athlete mind-set as its natural extension. Yogi Berra allegedly said that "sport is 50% physical and 90% mental." This is equally true of rehabilitation. Those who adhere only to the minimal criteria of rehabilitation progress slowly and haltingly. In contrast, those who bring emotional intensity modulated by a sensible and scientifically grounded knowledge base are most likely to make a remarkable recovery. Athletes are well-known for their absorption in what to outsiders may appear the minutiae of sport–subtle details of when and how to modify a technique to make it work better, better, and even better still. Those whose rehabilitation is complex or marked by setbacks need a similarly fine-tuned approach. By so doing, patient-athletes may relish the challenge of recovery and individualize their approach to rehabilitation in a way that best plays to their strengths while compensating for their weaknesses. In sum, the athlete mind-set is built on personal responsibility, a strong goal orientation, readiness to pursue physical training with intensity and precision, and a willingness to move one's physical and mental skills to a higher level of performance.

BRINGING PSYCHOLOGICAL MINDEDNESS
TO REHABILITATION

The established standard of care in the treatment of chronic pain emphasizes a multidisciplinary approach (Commission on the Accreditation of Rehabilitation Facilities, 1994). The core treatment team at a pain management center typically includes specialists in medicine, psychology, physical therapy, occupational therapy, and nursing. The state of the art in treatment is a carefully coordinated team approach which includes collaborative intervention and shared decision making. At our treatment center, we consider the patient a member of the treatment team as well. A strong goal-driven approach emphasizes consistency, careful pacing, and measured steady progress. Synergistic effects are noted as carefully coordinated cross-disciplinary interventions combine to collectively address specific problems. For example, habitual patterns of muscular guarding or bracing are commonly seen among chronic pain sufferers. This pattern of chronic muscle tension is typically maintained by a mutually reinforcing cycle of cause and effect. Fear of pain or reinjury may cause the patient to inhibit free movement of the injured area. This in turn may elicit chronic muscle tension and anxiety. This results in more pain as the individual tries to move an area of the body while paradoxically simultaneously protecting it. Guarding is best addressed simultaneously through the use of physical therapy modalities, therapeutic exercise, body mechanics, and self-regulation skills training to facilitate body awareness and reduced muscular tension.

Heil (1993) has synthesized behavioral medicine (that typically guides the treatment of chronic pain) with sport psychology to create a model of rehabilitation which helps turn patients into patient-athletes by fostering the development of the athlete mind-set. All treatment providers have an important role to play in the psychological management of the injured patient. In this model psychologists have equally important roles in the provision of both direct and indirect services. Direct services that are the exclusive province of psychology include psychological self-regulation skills training and cognitive behavioral therapies. In collaboration with the treatment team, the psychologist also works to enhance motivation via manipulation of behavioral contingencies and to manage resistance through behavioral contracting. These approaches have been thoroughly described by Fordyce (1976) and Turk, Meichenbaum, and Genest (1983). The reader is encouraged to consult these resources.

The goal of the psychologist as a provider of indirect services is to coach the other members of the treatment team to increase the psychological sophistication of their interventions. While medical providers have established psychologically relevant methods and practices, they are typically intuitively derived. Methods are usually taught anecdotally and through example, and learned by modeling mentors. The absence of a theoretical grounding and systematic instruction leaves these skills underdeveloped. The recently adopted *Role Delineation Study* of the National Athletic Training Association (1995), however, offers promise as a model for integrating psychological concepts and methods into rehabilitation.

The methods and skills which underlie what is colloquially regarded as "bedside manner" remain relatively undefined. From our perspective, the raw material of effective day-to-day patient management is education, goal-setting, and social support. The overall impact of medical intervention is enhanced as medical providers systematize and refine the psychological component of their treatment. As a team member, the psychologist can facilitate this process.

An equally important role for the psychologist is in leading the treatment team in troubleshooting compliance problems and managing treatment setbacks. The psychologist gathers relevant information from the treatment team, develops an intervention plan, guides providers in its implementation, then reassesses and modifies the plan as needed. Simultaneously, the psychologist has the opportunity to teach by example, modeling effective goal-setting and interpersonal problem-solving skills. Because problems present with urgency and immediacy and have direct impact on the ability of the medical providers to conduct their interventions, effective leadership by the psychologist is highly valued. Success in this arena demonstrates the value of psychology in medical interventions and offers the psychologist a proactive opportunity to integrate education, goal-setting and social support into medical treatments.

Effective use of education, goal setting, and social support begins with recognition of the critical role of psychology and a commitment to an egalitarian team approach. The foundation is laid through cross-disciplinary training as the psychologist and other providers share treatment concepts and assimilate knowledge outside the typical boundaries of their disciplines. Finally, these methods come to fruition as they are implemented formally in treatment planning and less formally in collaborative interactions between treatment providers.

Education is essential for the patient to understand the nature of the injury and the rehabilitation process. Table 1 lists an overview of topics for injury education. Through education, the patient becomes invested in the process of rehabilitation. This occurs as growth in knowledge creates a sense of confidence and mastery.

Whereas education provides the answer to the "what?" of rehabilitation, goal setting answers the question "how?" Goal setting across all treatments helps foster realistic expectations, encourages steady, consistent progress, and offers a realistically positive vision of the future. In essence, a carefully constructed program of goal setting creates a road map to recovery.

Social support is a subtle but potent influence on physical and mental well-being in injury and illness (Hardy & Crace, 1993; Sarason, Sarason &

TABLE 1. Injury Education Guidelines

Basic anatomy of the injured area

Physical changes caused by injury

Active and passive rehabilitation methods

Mechanisms by which rehabilitation methods work

Description of diagnostic and surgical procedures (if necessary)

Potential problems with pain and how to cope with these

Differentiation of benign pain from dangerous pain

Guidelines for independent use of modalities (i.e., heat, cold)

Plan for progressing active rehabilitation (e.g., resistance training)

Anticipated timetable for rehabilitation

Possibility of treatment plateaus

Purposes of medication with emphasis on consistent use as prescribed

Potential side effects of medication with encouragement to report these to the physician

Rationale for limits on daily physical activities during healing

Guidelines for the use of braces, orthotic devices, and crutches

Injury as a source of stress and a challenge to maintaining a positive attitude

Rehabilitation as an active collaborative learning process

Methods of assessing readiness for return to play

Deciding when to hold back and when to go all-out

Long-term maintenance and care of healing injury

Pierce, 1990). Treatment providers are key players in the patient's support network. The more severe the injury and the more isolated the patient-athlete is from his or her usual environment, the more critical the social support from treatment providers becomes. All members of the treatment team offer critical emotional support in order to help the patient-athlete through his or her weakest moments. As the team members observe the athlete make important steps forward and triumph over challenge, they are also able to recognize and reinforce effort given and mastery achieved. Trust in the treatment team helps the patient athlete overcome the anxieties innate to medical environments, as well as the fear of reinjury and other concerns which may serve as barriers to successful rehabilitation. World Cup skier Christin Cooper offers an insightful perspective on the psychological impact of her physician orthopaedic surgeon, Richard Steadman. She describes

> arriving on his doorstep as a scared and impatient 16-year-old with a badly broken ankle. I expected surgery and ended up . . . learning things from Steadman that went beyond the operating room–about ourselves, our injuries, and our sport . . . Steadman creates a psychological profile and determines . . . the exact ratio between surgery and exercise, inspiration and rehab. (Cooper, 1992, pp. 181-183)

SPORT PSYCHOLOGY IN REHABILITATION

For the psychologist working with medical populations, behavioral medicine skills are a fundamental prerequisite. The behavioral medicine specialist can refine intervention strategies to optimize injury rehabilitation by incorporating the principles and practices of sport psychology. This section focuses on the transfer of sport psychology techniques to rehabilitation, as well as the benefits of interacting with the patient-athlete on site in the rehabilitation setting.

The hallmark of sport psychology has been the development of mental skills training to improve performance in competitive environments. These methods are essentially adaptations of cognitive behavioral techniques modified to develop the mental skills upon which athletic performance depends. Mental training often relies on intricate mental rehearsal strategies that incorporate methods for refining concentration and decision making in response to specific challenges. For a thorough review of varied mental training methods, sport specific goal-setting and other sport psychology techniques, see Henschen and Straub (1995) or Van Raalte and Brewer (1996). While it is beyond the scope of this paper to deal with mental training in detail, an application of mental rehearsal to rehabilitation will be briefly described.

Mental rehearsal techniques can be used to help athletes anticipate and deal with the challenges of rehabilitation. This approach may be used in the early stages of treatment in anticipation of a particularly challenging course of rehabilitation or if early signs of potential adjustment problems are noted. Alternately, this rehearsal method may be used during later stages of rehabilitation in response to specific problems. The psychologist and patient-athlete collaborate to construct a rehearsal scenario that identifies a specific rehabilitation problem as the athlete sees it. It is embellished with multisensory language that elaborates the sights, sounds, and kinesthetic feel of the activity. For example, consider the patient-athlete who periodically experiences brief anxious episodes in response to the slow and protracted nature of rehabilitation. A strategy is devised which begins with the patient-athlete practicing relaxation procedures to create a calming stress management effect and set the stage for mental rehearsal. Then the athlete calls to mind the problem situation in enough detail to create the feeling of being there. This is followed by a rehearsal of selected coping methods, such as deep breathing, positive imagery, and self-talk which cultivate a positive attitude. Heil (1993) offers an in-depth description of mental training methods in injury rehabilitation.

Of great importance for the true integration of psychologists into the treatment team is their presence in the treatment environment. Just as sport psychologists routinely educate themselves about the sports of the athletes with whom they work, so knowledge of physical rehabilitation must be assimilated to gain efficacy as a treatment provider. Seeing rehabilitation in action is the best way to gain an appreciation of the subtleties and nuances of therapeutic exercise, aerobic conditioning, sport and work skills. Being on-site allows the psychologist to sample patient behavior outside the clinical office, precisely where the challenge is unfolding. This offers the opportunity to observe the extent to which attitudes and behaviors essential to treatment success are operative in the rehabilitation setting and facilitates timely reinforcement of effort and gains in physical performance. In addition, the psychologist is better able to assess and address barriers to effective rehabilitation. Finally, being on-site allows for a more effective collaborative effort among team members by providing an ideal setting for treatment planning and the exchange of cross-disciplinary knowledge.

CASE STUDY

The following case study illustrates the synthesis of sport psychology and behavioral medicine and its integration into a multidisciplinary chronic pain treatment program. Myrna is a 35-year-old female with arm and back pain. She was referred by her orthopaedic physician to the Pain Management Center where she underwent multidisciplinary evaluation by medicine, psychology, occupational therapy and physical therapy. The patient's history, treatment plan, and treatment summary appear below.

History

Myrna was injured in a motor vehicle accident approximately seven months prior to her evaluation. Because of soreness and difficulty using her right arm, as well as lower back and mid-back pain, she was seen in an emergency room. Evaluation showed no fracture or neurologic injury. She was prescribed medicines and referred to an orthopaedic physician. Problems with her right arm continued as her back pain increased. A course of physical therapy met with mixed success. She experienced anxiety while driving in the period immediately following her motor vehicle accident, but this had gradually resolved over time.

Myrna struggled unsuccessfully to return to work and to resume her sport and routine household activities. Myrna had been employed at a medium to heavy work task that required overtime. Prior to injury she raised horses and regularly competed in dressage events. She described increased pain with prolonged sitting or standing, bending and lifting–all of which were required on the job and at home. The bouncing, jarring effects of horseback riding also increased her pain and led her to discontinue riding. Myrna was using narcotic analgesic medicines on an ongoing basis. Unsuccessful attempts at return to work and horseback riding were followed with increased medication use which resulted in narcotic dependence.

Myrna described feelings of loss over her inability to work, ride her horse, and maintain her household. She was experiencing mild depression with frustration, irritability, and moodiness. She also complained of fatigue and difficulty with concentration. Sleep had become increasingly restless with delay in sleep onset and regular nocturnal awakenings.

Treatment Plan

Multidisciplinary pain evaluation failed to identify neurologic injury or other condition requiring surgery or acute medical treatment. Because of the entrenched and progressive nature of her pain, pervasive lifestyle disruption, and growing depression, an intensive team approach to rehabilitation was recommended. Her treatment plan was developed based on the results of the initial evaluation and on Myrna's statement of personal goals. The plan was then reviewed with Myrna and revised based on her comments. In the process, personal responsibility was implicitly emphasized as educational concepts were introduced and the central role of goal setting was identified. The team treatment plan is summarized in Table 2.

Treatment Summary

Myrna completed a multidisciplinary rehabilitation program that included ongoing medical evaluation and medication management, physical therapy and occupational therapy, as well as individual and group psychotherapy. Direct psychological services included clarification of the patient's understanding of the concepts underlying pain, injury, and rehabilitation; normalizing the sense of loss and feelings of anxiety that accompany injury and rehabilitation; and training in self-regulation and other cognitive behavioral skills to manage stress, pain, sleep, and other psychological sequelae. For Myrna in particular, emphasis was placed on approaching rehabilitation as a workout and on bringing the physical precision that characterized her riding to a wide range of work and other day-to-day activities.

Treatment was conducted in two phases. The initial intensive phase took place three days a week over a period of six weeks (approximately 20 hours per week) at the Pain Management Center and was supplemented by home exercise programs. It was designed to teach basic rehabilitation skills and to create positive psychological momentum. In a subsequent follow-up program, Myrna met with treatment team members at two-week intervals (about one half day's duration) for a period of three months. The follow-up program was designed to continue skill development and to guide Myrna in generalizing skills to an increasing array of activities. Her responsibility for implementing the treatment plan grew as the frequency and intensity of supervision decreased. Because of her athletic background, there was a focus on transfer of existing sport knowledge and skills to rehabilitation.

During the initial week of treatment, Myrna was hesitant regarding physical interventions and mildly skeptical of psychological treatment. Her readiness to proceed with treatment and sense of hope were cultivated through discussion of the general conditioning principles used in training horses and the transferability of these principles to her own rehabilitation. Psychological treatment was presented as a means of refining skills in goal setting, improving concentration and sleep, and managing irritability. During the second week of treatment, therapeutic exercise and aerobic exercise programs began in earnest. The physical and occupational therapist called Myrna's attention to the natural grace and fluidity of her horse and

TABLE 2. Lewis-Gale Pain Center Admission Treatment Plan

Patient Name: Myrna   Case Manager: Jackson Metcalf

PROBLEM LIST WITH ACCOMPANYING GOALS OF TREATMENT

1. Diminished Coping
       Poor Pain Tolerance
       Stress
       Sleep Disturbance
       Short-Term Goals: Improve pain/stress knowledge
                              Improve pain/stress management skills
                              Demonstrate ability to manage pain flare-ups, using
                                 appropriate techniques
                              Improve sleep quality (duration/onset/awakenings)
       Long-Term Goals: Maintain skills in pain/stress management generalizing
                                 to an increasing array of activities and situations
                              Maintain healthy sleep patterns without medication
                              Improve pain tolerance
2. Pain
       Pain Varying Under Diverse Circumstances
       Short-Term Goals: Report symptoms appropriately within treatment setting
       Long-Term Goals: Decrease pain report overall
                              Report decreased pain with specific activities of daily living
3. Diminished Psychological Status
       Pain Behaviors (body language and/or vocal)
       Depressive Dysphoria
       Situational Anxiety
       Short-Term Goals: Decrease pain behaviors (across varied conditions)
                              Decrease situational anxiety
                              Decrease depressive dysphoria
       Long-Term Goals: Stabilize and enhance gains in mood
                              Continue to decrease pain behaviors
4. Medication Use
       Narcotic Analgesic Reliance
       Short-Term Goals: Discontinue narcotic analgesic medication
                              Comply with recommended medication use to
                                 manage pain and sleep
       Long-Term Goals: Maintenance of appropriate medication regimen
                                 to manage symptoms

TABLE 2 (continued)

5. Diminished Physical Capacity
        Postural Deviations
        Decreased Flexibility
        Decreased Strength
        Decreased Endurance
        Poor Body Mechanics
        Problems with Walking/Gait
        Inability to Perform Work Tasks
        Inability to Perform Sport–Horseback Riding
        Decreased Social/Leisure Activities
        Inability to Perform Home Tasks

    Short-Term Goals: Demonstrate improved static/dynamic posture
                         Movements performed in smooth coordinated
                            fashion with decreased pain/compensatory
                            movements
                         Perform safe aerobic activity progressing toward
                            target heart rate (3-5 times a week)
                         Display improved gait pattern, improved speed/distance
                         Follow through with home exercise program
                            when not in attendance at Pain Center
                         Improve sit and stand tolerance

    Long-Term Goals: Demonstrate flexibility/strength/endurance
                            sufficient to perform all activities of daily living
                         Demonstrate appropriate use of body mechanics/
                            joint protection/work simplification/problem-solving
                            with work, sport, and other activities of daily living
                         Progressive return to gainful employment
                         Gradual resumption of horseback riding
                         Perform premorbid level leisure/social activities
                         Perform premorbid level of other activities of
                            daily living
                         Independently/consistently perform home exercise
                            program
                         Maintain/increase gains in posture/flexibility/
                            strength/endurance

herself as a rider–and encouraged her to bring the same smooth efficient movements to her exercise and daily activities. Narcotic analgesic medicines were tapered over the next two weeks of treatment with the patient continuing to use acetaminophen only for pain. Simultaneously, she was prescribed a non-habit-forming medicine to help manage sleep. Psychological treatment addressed coping with loss and developing the athlete mind-set to prepare Myrna for the challenge of the prolonged course of rehabilitation she faced. Over subsequent weeks, Myrna continued to progress in treatment with gradual gains in physical ability and psychological coping skills. At the conclusion of the intensive treatment phase, all range-of-motion and strength measures were improved. Regular compliance with her aerobic program had led to notable increases in endurance. A specialized gait training program dramatically improved walking. Steady improvement was noted in psychological status. Initial gains in energy and concentration were followed by decreased moodiness and irritability. Sleep gradually improved over time with the eventual taper of sleep medicine. Psychological intervention focused on understanding the interrelationship of pain, physical function, and psychological state as well as continued skill building. During the last two weeks of treatment, Myrna returned to work on a part-time, light duty basis. She gradually progressed to full-time work with slightly modified duties. By the conclusion of intensive treatment, she was able to resume most household and leisure activities.

Because of the entrenched nature of chronic pain, treatment seldom proceeds simply and continually on course. Treatment setbacks challenge providers to function as a team and call for leadership from the psychologist. For example, Myrna met with a significant set-back in her horseback riding shortly after she began the follow-up component of the treatment program. She had gradually and successfully resumed riding. During the intensive phase of treatment, Myrna experienced a sudden pain flare-up when her horse made a sudden awkward movement during her initial attempt to ride with moderate intensity. She lost control of her horse briefly before dismounting and walking the horse back to the barn. She continued to work but with some restrictions added for a limited time. Horseback riding was discontinued, as were a variety of household activities. Physical symptoms resolved rather slowly with gradual increase in work and household activities. However, Myrna appeared to be more depressed, exhibiting a subtle yet uncharacteristic sense of hopelessness and apathy. Her rehabilitation, now conducted for the most part independently, was less vigorous and consistent. In addition, she was now anxious about and reluctant to resume riding. In the interview, it became apparent that this incident had elicited doubts about whether she would be able to return to her prior level of competitive ability and had undermined her self-confidence. The treatment team collaborated to create a goal-directed plan for return to riding, emphasizing proper posture and body mechanics with extended warm-up and cool-down. A psychological intervention program focused on reducing specific fears of reinjury and generalized anxiety regarding pain with routine riding.

A thought-stopping program was implemented to manage negative thoughts regarding self-confidence and fear of reinjury. This was supplemented by a refocusing strategy that emphasized tuning in to the rhythm of the horse. Myrna gradually resumed her riding and regained her confidence. By the time the final phase of treatment had been concluded, she was planning to return to competition.

Overview

By cultivating personal responsibility, building a knowledge base regarding pain and rehabilitation, demonstrating effective goal setting, and challenging her to approach rehabilitation as an athlete, Myrna was able to break the cycle of chronic pain. Gradually, the trauma of her injury was diminished and she was able to regain a satisfying quality of life.

CONCLUSION

The case of Myrna illustrates how an injured recreational athlete can optimize her recovery by drawing on the principles of sport and physical training. It also demonstrates the benefits of coaching from the treatment team in the cultivation of the athlete mind-set. We contend that a similar approach to intervention is broadly applicable to rehabilitation with appropriate modification to accommodate the level of athleticism the patient brings to treatment. The patient-athlete metaphor is conceptually rich and intrinsically appealing to patients and treatment providers. It offers a perspective from which to understand the challenges of rehabilitation and the skills upon which recovery depends.

REFERENCES

Berryman, J. W. (1995). *Out of many, one: A history of the American College of Sportsmedicine.* Champaign, IL: Human Kinetics.

Bonica, J. J. (1991). Pain management: Past and current status including role of the anesthesiologist. In T. H. Stanley, M.A. Ashburn & P. G. Fine (Eds.), *Anesthesiology and pain management* (pp. 1-30). Boston: Kiuwer.

Bozoian, S., Rejeski, W. J., & McAuley, E. (1994). Self-efficacy influences feeling states associated with acute exercise. *Journal of Sport & Exercise Psychology, 16* (3), 326-333.

Browne, M. A. & Mahoney, M. G. (1994). Sport psychology. *Annual Review of Psychology 35, 605-625.*

Commission on Accreditation of Rehabilitation Facilities. (1994). *Standards manual and interpretive guidelines for organizations serving people with disabilities.* Tucson, AZ: Author.

Cooper, Christin (1992, November). Steadie. *Skiing 45*(3), pp. 180-182, 185, 187-188, 272.

Dolce, J. J., Crocker, M. F., Moleteire, C., & Doleys, D. M. (1986). Exercise quotas, anticipatory concern and self-efficacy expectancies in chronic pain: A preliminary report. *Pain 24,* 365-372.

Druckman, A. & Bjork, R. A. (Eds.). (1991). *In the minds' eye: Enhancing human performance.* Washington, DC: National Academy Press.

Fordyce, W. (1976). *Behavioral methods for chronic pain and illness.* St. Louis: Mosby.

Fordyce, W., McMahon, R., Rainwater, G., Jackins, S., Questad, K., Murphy, T., & DeLateur, B. (1981). Pain compliant–exercise performance relationship in chronic pain. *Pain, 10,* 311-321.

Hardy, C. J. & Crace, R. K. (1993). The dimensions of social support when dealing with sport injuries. In D. Pargman (Ed.), *Psychological bases of sport injuries* (pp. 121-144). Morgantown, WV: Fitness Information Technology.

Heil, J. (1993). *Psychology of sport injury.* Champaign, IL: Human Kinetics.

Henschen, K. P., & Straub, W. F. (Eds.). (1995). *Sport psychology: An analysis of athlete behavior* (3rd ed.). Longmeadow, MA: Mouvement.

Ievleva, L., & Orlick, T. (1991). Mental links to enhanced healing: An exploratory study. *The Sport Psychologist. 5(1),* 25-40.

Long, B. C., & Van Stravel, R. (1995). Effects of exercise training on anxiety: A meta-analysis. *Journal of Applied Sport Psychology. 1,* 167-189.

National Athletics Training Association (1995). *Role Delineation Study: The National Athletic Training Association Board of Certification. Inc. Third Edition.* Philadelphia: F.A. Davis.

Nicoloff, G. & Schwenk, T. L. (1995). Using exercise to ward off depression. *The Physician and Sportsmedicine,* 23(9), 44-46, 51-52, 55-57.

Orlick, T. (1990). *In pursuit of excellence.* Champaign, IL: Human Kinetics.

Ravizza, X. (1988). Gaining entry with athletic personnel for season-long consulting. *The Sport Psychologist, 2(3),* 243-254.

Sarason, B. R., Sarason, I. G., Pierce, G. R. (Eds.). (1990). *Social support: An interactional view.* New York: Wiley.

Steadman, J. R. (1982). Rehabilitation of skiing injuries. *Clinics in Sportsmedicine 1* (2), 289-294.

Turk, D. C., Meichenbaum, D., & Genest, M. (1983). *Pain and behavioral medicine: A cognitive behavioral perspective.* New York: Guilford Press.

Van Raalte, J. L. & Brewer, B. N. (Eds.). (1996). *Exploring sport and exercise psychology.* Washington, DC: American Psychological Association.

Weinberg, R. S. & Gould, D. (Eds.). (1995). *Foundations of sport and exercise psychology.* Champaign, IL: Human Kinetics.

Williams, R.C. (1995, December). Estimating costs of chronic pain syndrome. Workshop on selected chronic pain conditions: clinical spectrum, frequency and costs, sponsored by the National Institute of Health Interagency Task Force on Chronic Pain, Bethesda, MD.

Contact Improvisation:
Its Potentials
for a Therapy of Movement:
A Conversation/Dialogue Between
Nancy Menapace and E. Mark Stern

Nancy Menapace
E. Mark Stern

E. Mark Stern: Nancy, you're involved in Contact Improvisation (referred to throughout this interview as "CI"), a unique dance format with possible therapeutic implications. Let's begin with your own history in CI.

Nancy Menapace: I started in a class in contact skills taught by Andrew Harwood at the Bates College Dance Festival in Maine. This was followed by more advanced work at the Naropa Institute in Boulder, Colorado. It was there that I learned more of how CI engages two partners in dance, beginning with gestures, moving into simple touch, and eventually into intense physical engagement. Full body contact, aimed at a sharing of mutual weight, becomes a unique aesthetic goal.

CI, as a dance form, became a performance constituent of the then Judson Church dance movement in 1972. Judson Church, located on

---

Nancy Menapace, a graduate of George Washington University, is currently teaching yoga and stretch in Washington, DC.

E. Mark Stern, EdD, ABPP, is Professor Emeritus at Iona College and a clinical psychologist in private practice in New York City.

[Haworth co-indexing entry note]: "Contact Improvisation: Its Potentials for a Therapy of Movement: A Conversation/Dialogue Between Nancy Menapace and E. Mark Stern." Menapace, Nancy, and E. Mark Stern. Co-published simultaneously in *The Psychotherapy Patient* (The Haworth Press, Inc.) Vol. 10, No. 3/4, 1998, pp. 41-46; and: *Integrating Exercise, Sports, Movement and Mind: Therapeutic Unity* (ed: Kate F. Hays) The Haworth Press, Inc., 1998, pp. 41-46. Single or multiple copies of this article are available for a fee from The Haworth Document Delivery Service [1-800-342-9678, 9:00 a.m. - 5:00 p.m. (EST). E-mail address: getinfo@haworth.com].

41

Washington Square South in New York's Greenwich Village, has historically provided performance space and encouragement to the emerging arts. Steve Paxton, Nancy Stark Smith, and Danny Lebkov were the primary figures in CI's history and development. I guess Steve Paxton stands as the founder and the other two as primary motivators. As far as I know, Steve Paxton is living in Vermont and still exploring movements in dance. Other dimensions of the work have been taking place at Oberlin College in Ohio which, along with Judson Church, had early become a center for CI exploration and training.

EMS: So CI, a dance form, expands on the possibilities for artistic expressiveness?

NM: Right. Imagine a simple dance, involving two people, whose expressive repertoire emerges as they touch each other's fingertips. As the exploration goes on, they might introduce their hands to one another. Eventually whole arms and torsos meet. The dance becomes aerial. And it is here that the possibility of "shared weight" takes form. The momentum of the two bodies meeting leads into a full momentum of contact. Then, just as easily as it all began, the partners return to the initial motif of two fingertips touching and parting.

EMS: The sharing of weight then becomes a joint negotiation?

NM: Yes. It is the product of gesture and movement.

EMS: It sounds like a metaphor for equality?

NM: Precisely. A momentum is initiated. As the process develops, each person takes the lead. First one dancer, then the other, *initiates a new idea of the form.* When I'm involved in the dance, I am not beholden to either leading or following. What I do experience is finding myself groping at survival positions. If I fail to go with the momentum, I can likely hurt myself. I must remain resolutely alert in order to avoid falling on my head. I refer to the dance relationship in terms of weight. This means that I sometimes take the lead, sometimes not. But always the nature of the dance is to share the weight. Ideally, no one leads or follows. Aeriness becomes the byproduct of subtle shifts in the distribution of weight. A dancer may freely take the other's weight in order to allow an air move in which the one dancer flies for both of them. Sometimes a dancer will want to fly alone. This means not assuming positions suggestive of taking the other's weight. The standards of excellence are the felt negotiations where both remain in control and not in control in different ways.

EMS: CI paradigms would appear to be useful in the psychotherapy process since dance metaphors certainly relate well to the world of words. When either patient or therapist initiates, the words become "induced movement" (after Duncker, cited by Wolfgang Kohler, 1947). Like two trains, the one moving and the other stationary, each person seems to be coordinated in taking an equal direction. Perhaps they have etched out a position of sharing weight?

NM: That's it. Sharing weight happens when two figures can be jointly defined. The CI dance takes place when each of the participants feels comfortable with his or her specific strengths. What's nice about CI is that when the dancers are involved, controls move to the side. Movement is happening so quickly. One freely gives as the other equally takes weight. Who's in control isn't even a question. It's all so fluid.

EMS: In the verbal dance of psychotherapy, weight, too, becomes a necessary illusion. Metaphors reign. The weight of disclosure corresponds with the weight of interpretation. The humanistic psychologist's emphasis on therapist selective self-disclosure becomes foundational for radically egalitarian shifts of weight. Both parties to the therapeutic enterprise are best appreciated through their dynamic flux.

NM: I agree. It's the capacity to see processes in transition. There are many possibilities for the development of aerie (freely giving and freely taking) relationships. If I give in to the temptation of self-navigating the dance, its range becomes severely restricted. *Throwing* my weight around makes for something limited and boring. On the other hand, where one dancer consistently feels it necessary to seize control, the dance itself can begin to serve as its own corrective. It's amazing how in these circumstances both dancers are alerted to the implausibility of one of them sustaining uninterrupted control. Contact assumes shared weight. Therefore, CI tends to transform both parties into a recognition of each other's necessity.

EMS: Can mere symmetry mimic airiness?

NM: I doubt it. Being in the dance fosters its own culture; one that encourages participants to share. If there's going to be any pressure at all, it's going to be in trying to be equal. The cultural emphasis makes a plea for striving for that equality as a way of discovering authentic power.

EMS: So it's the shifting between active and passive positions which fosters good practice both in CI and in the psychotherapeutic discourse.

I'm reminded of Rollo May's (1969) relating Mozart's rotating quintets to pure sensuous pleasure. In psychotherapy, rotation is not simply a way of reversing roles. Rather than a mere gathering of verbal connections, psychotherapy evokes emergent epiphanies made of new and unique experiential arrangements. As the "weight" of therapist and patient is finally shared, as egalitarianism is encouraged, so, too, are futility and disenfranchisement reversed. Each of the parties to the therapeutic project is freed to enjoy the results of a newly established hardiness and hopefulness.

NM: What I most enjoy about CI is observing expressive language. Observation helps me appreciate how my partner dancer could go further. When I see a holding back by placing certain limits on expression, I'm in a position to approach in my partner's dance style. I can play, and in that play with my partner, I can be part of the inauguration of expansion, moving to places which reveal where we really want to be, but are somewhat fearful of approaching.

EMS: Sharing power or weight become explicit goals. Is it here that a particular sort of person is attracted to the ethos within the dance?

NM: Interestingly, most practitioners of CI have had little if any background in athletics or specifically in gymnastics or dance. People are drawn by the spontaneity of the dance jams.

EMS: Somewhat like musicians being attracted to jazz jams?

NM: Probably. They're not necessarily experienced dancers. The jams attract a broad range of people from computer scientists to environmentalists. There are varying numbers in any one jam. In Washington, we have anywhere from five to twenty participants at a time.

EMS: What are the agreed-on terms?

NM: Jams open with everyone finding a place in a circle. Everyone has the opportunity to exchange verbal thoughts and feelings. Some jams center around a particular exploratory theme, which acts as a springboard into dancing. But even without a focus, each participant is free to decide on a person to dance with. Likewise, participants are free to choose not to dance.

EMS: What I recall when observing a CI performance was that dancers may bring a constricted or expansive view of space and movement to the task. Even though, as you say, backgrounds appear to matter less as determinants, I'd be interested in knowing how your particular dance background has mattered to you?

NM: I think I'm an exception. I had an extended competitive gymnastics background. The experience has been helpful because I already had a freedom in my sense of movement through space when I came to CI. I knew how to fall because I've been trained to have a very strong sense of self-possession. I was able to step in with a certain freedom, at least physically. But, like others, I had much to learn through participation with partners.

EMS: It's no secret that you've been wanting to integrate CI into some area of movement therapy or physical therapy. How do you envision CI as a force in the healing arts?

NM: I'm pleasantly naive above the attitudes of movement therapists. But I do know about psychotherapy. I've experienced it and those experiences have furthered my belief that CI has the potential of being most profound in providing insight.

EMS: Are you differentiating between insights fostered in CI and those found in verbal psychotherapy?

NM: Since I meet so many different people, I'm continually challenged and stimulated by their respective ways of handling life situations. In CI people leave it to physical language. There is little or no discussion of sexuality, or of other emotional aspects of what's going on interpersonally. In a way this is very freeing, but it can also limit things. This may be changing. At the jams, everything begins and ends with the circles. Participants are free to open up discussions of what it feels like or felt like to be in a certain dance, aspects of the actions which are liked or disliked. This opens the dialogue in ways unique to feeling through physical expression.

EMS: The therapeutic potentialities inherent in CI open up new metaphors for change. Invitation, engagement, and initiation become exciting possibilities.

NM: Definitely. But physical dialogue between people has always been like a dance. People may be more *aware* than they have the immediate capacity to be conscious of. Gestalt Therapy says as much. It, like CI, fosters physical positioning and absurdity as means of helping people change. The combination of both techniques has provided me with a means of transforming my physical and psychological patterns. I think CI can be helpful both on its own and within the context and language of any number of therapeutic schools of thought. The final consideration for CI must always be "Who is this person?" and "Why is he or she approaching and avoiding like this?" and finally, "What meaning does the dance confer on the dancers?"

REFERENCES

Kohler, W. (1947). *Gestalt psychology.* New York: New American Library.
May, R. (1969). *Love and will.* New York: W. W. Norton.

The Dialogue of Movement:
An Interview/Conversation
with Ilene Serlin
and E. Mark Stern

Ilene Serlin
E. Mark Stern

INTERVIEWER'S INTRODUCTION

I decided to interview Dr. Ilene Serlin because of her talents as a dance therapist. Dance therapy is a highly expressive body-focussed adjunct to psychotherapy. Yet as a psychotherapeutic discipline in its own right, dance therapy aims at the awakening and cultivation of a keen appreciation of the ways in which the client moves. Dance therapists, as a group, assume that people are only partially aware of themselves and then only as they concentrate and talk. The intention of dance therapy is to further advance an awareness of body moods. It employs and recognizes sad dances, happy dances, sensual dances and dances that signal others to keep a safe distance. Dance therapy concentrates on appreciating, and, where appropriate, changing sensory and emotional patternings. The discipline focuses on the interaction of bodies, the body's relationship to the environment, and the cultivation of emotional insight while the body is at rest or in deliberate or spontaneous motion.

Ilene Serlin, PhD, is affiliated with the Saybrook Institute, San Francisco, CA.
E. Mark Stern, EdD, ABPP, is Professor Emeritus at Iona College and a clinical psychologist in private practice in New York City.

[Haworth co-indexing entry note]: "The Dialogue of Movement: An Interview/Conversation with Ilene Serlin and E. Mark Stern." Serlin, Ilene, and E. Mark Stern. Co-published simultaneously in *The Psychotherapy Patient* (The Haworth Press, Inc.) Vol. 10, No. 3/4, 1998, pp. 47-52; and: *Integrating Exercise, Sports, Movement and Mind: Therapeutic Unity* (ed: Kate F. Hays) The Haworth Press, Inc., 1998, pp. 47-52. Single or multiple copies of this article are available for a fee from The Haworth Document Delivery Service [1-800-342-9678, 9:00 a.m. - 5:00 p.m. (EST). E-mail address: getinfo@haworth.com].

47

Dance therapists are trained in a variety of settings. Most have earned a master's level degree from institutions such as Leslie College in Cambridge, Massachusetts or the Pratt Institute in Brooklyn, New York. Others, with prior credentials in one of the mental health fields, go on to add dance therapy to their professional resources through continuing education workshops. And then there are accomplished dancers who have developed dance therapy skills through mentorships with psychotherapists and master dance therapists as well as on the scene activities in mental hospitals, rehabilitation centers, and special education settings to name but a few of the settings. Dr. Serlin, who is a trained licensed clinical psychologist, is a professor at the Saybrook Institute in San Francisco. She is also qualified as a dance therapist. And so the dialogue begins:

E. Mark Stern: I'm curious: How do you keep sight of boundaries in your work? More importantly, how do you manage to work within the boundaries which provide the space you require in dance therapy?

Ilene Serlin: Let me begin by commenting on how I see boundaries, and how problematic their acknowledgment becomes. It's a joke among dance therapists that we are better at merging than at separating. Still the structure of good therapy is built of strengths and weaknesses. We're trained kinesthetically to empathize, so that we are able to move in rhythm with the other. Therefore, the whole issue of boundaries is how *not* to get merged with the other. There are several means to accomplish this. One is that the dance therapist's personal verbal and/or movement psychotherapy helps in her or his knowing the differences between what's the "you" and what's the "other." This can only happen after knowing what it means to intuit the other. As a consequence of the practitioner feeling the other so intensely, the question of boundaries is even more powerful than it might be in the more usual psychotherapeutic encounter. Kinesthetic countertransferences are established in the presence of the other. Countertransference, when understood, provides the therapist with the means of distinguishing what's "mine" from what belongs to the other person. Obviously the client needs to be experienced on many levels. I see this as the strength of the process. Ensnaring traps along the way are potential weaknesses which require moment-to-moment reflectiveness. How else is one able to make the necessary discriminations for good therapy to take place?

EMS: Please give me an example of moment-to-moment therapeutic discriminations.

IS: Somebody comes into my office who I sense is in need of mothering. I feel that "need" in my own body. It may take the form of a desire to enfold, to make safe, to put my arms around the person and so forth. I now have to gauge how much of a comforting voice to use and how to mediate/ moderate what is and is not "motherly." My attention focuses on the maternal archetype which I often feel in my whole bearing and demeanor. Much of what happens is consummated in how I manage these feelings; how I become conscious of what is being constellated in the relationship. Based on this kind of information, I aim to work with sufficient attachment as well as detachment.

EMS: People who are in need of help are capable of provoking all sorts of feelings in the therapist. Earlier you alluded to kinesthetic countertransference as a physical sensitivity to what the client is trying to express. What's your impression of how the client reacts to your feelings?

IS: Let me speak from the complexity of the question itself. Suppose I am feeling degrees of maternal sensibility. Could these sensations be some way of being called forth as a comforting presence? It is my responsibility to attempt to discern whether, in that moment, what the client truly wants is growth producing. Or is the client simply in need of a safe place, and in that state of need, playing with old patterns? I must try to be clear whether what I see as a need for nearness is possibly fostering claustrophobia. In other words, my first felt inclination to offer safety may not be what is most needed. So how to discriminate between what is regressive and what is helpful? My moment-to-moment decisions on how to move become quite consequential for that person. I must always ask myself, am I being asked to help reinforce what has been stifled and restricted in the past, or is the request a means of calling forth satisfaction of that which had never been there for the client in the past?

EMS: What is it that makes you feel you "know"?

IS: There are so many streams of information coming in at any given moment. I come to each situation with a rich background of experiences which inform me of what may be subtly taking place. I have learned the dangers of overprotecting even those who ask for it, while at the same time, I've come to appreciate my way of searching for what is most appropriate for one person and not another.

EMS: On several occasions in the late 1950s, I was given the opportunity of observing Dr. John Rosen, then of the Department of Psychiatry of Temple University, work with a pioneering approach to psychotherapy with chronic psychotics he dubbed "Direct Analysis." His patients were all withdrawn schizophrenics who were in residences in Doylestown, Pennsylvania. Each patient lived in a separate cottage shared with a staff of "assistant therapists." Dr. Rosen's interventions were certainly intensive. He rarely hesitated being verbally and physically confrontive and encouraged the same in round-the-clock therapy by his assistants. In "entering" the "worlds" of his patients, Dr. Rosen described himself as their "mother." This gave him permission to feed them, soothe them, and plead with them for a relationship. There were times that he used shaming devices and on at least one occasion wrestled a man down to the floor. His dedication to addressing the primary processes he assumed were active in his patients was amazing to watch. From what I saw of his work, and in two subsequent published interchanges with him, I knew that his particular style was unique. Even more so when he declared that, "so much of the mother have I become that the day I 'kick-off' (i.e., die), most of my cured patients will revert back to psychosis because of the separation that they felt in their infancies." I should mention that the bulk of his assistant therapists were people he described as his former now ex-psychotic patients. It's no wonder that my ears perk up when you speak of embracing the mother archetype in psychotherapy. Perhaps you do something other than what Dr. Rosen did. For one, you do not work with a primarily psychotic population. And from my knowing you, it's obvious that you try to give the client ample room to develop his or her own strategies. Why don't you amplify your notions of mothering in the dance therapy process?

IS: I've studied films made by the late anthropologist Margaret Mead which illustrate the centrality of cradling infants. Cradling points to a need for containment. The impulse to cradle is something I readily feel in my work. People are scattered and unable to focus in their lives. They need containment to assist them in prioritizing. In other words people who are lacking in the capacity to contain are hardly aware of their feet falling. A therapeutic ideal is to help these clients spatially contain themselves. There is a caution, namely that the dance therapist, in the process of motherly containing, doesn't inadvertently crowd in or squeeze. People may react negatively to the slightest feeling of pressure. There is a sort of holding space somewhere between too much and too little. It's beneficial to hold and offer steadiness, but not to the point of diminishing or controlling the client. On the other hand, it is sometimes unsatisfactory to diffuse a hold if the client is liable to fall. There must be a balance between freedom and feeling safe. Good therapy aims at providing enough safety in which the client is able to feel freedom. This doesn't necessarily imply touch. I may at times sit with the client. The best way to illustrate is to examine the way I may inhabit the space, and the way I surround the person in the expanse we make together.

EMS: Do the clients who call on you for dance therapy necessarily know how to dance?

IS: Some have been specifically referred for dance therapy. Many do not know how to dance. Others who were referred for verbal therapy get the benefit of the way I sense their expressive energy through the archetypal sensibilities that flow through me. It may *look* to an observer as if we are just sitting and talking. Dance therapy clients have the opportunity of seeing the images in a more externalized way. Dance can be about closeness, apartness, small and big and so forth. Dance therapy physicalizes these emotions. As soon as the client enters my space, we begin to play out these affective states.

EMS: What do you mean by "play them out?"

IS: It's a matter of what the client is open for.

EMS: What it is to feel like receiving?

IS: Absolutely. I recall a client whose central concern was about being diminished. We entered into an improvised dance in which she was sinking and becoming smaller. This alternated by gestures of being bigger and bigger. As she sank and became smaller, I made very big gestures. As she followed my lead, I made sure to take on smaller dimensions. Allowing her to find what was comfortable helped her to understand how she made people bigger or smaller than life. I tend to use polarities as constructions to emphasize a theme. Near and far can trigger many issues. It is existential, since the process of dance therapy becomes a slow motion picture framed within the client's view of his or her time/space lived in world. Dance as a play form becomes an essential means of experiencing appropriateness. My role as therapist rests with helping the client understand when "near" or "far" threatens. Obviously early memories come into play when nearness and distance are so intimately experienced.

EMS: How do you sense that these memories are becoming activated?

IS: Sometimes verbally, but at other times, kinesthetically, that is in movements expressing quick/slow; big/little; near/far. Becoming sensitive to the underlying history and context of the client's emotional life is important to the development of diagnostic skills. I must emphasize that I try to stay closest to characteristic/characterological structures which trigger themselves beyond what the client may have verbally reported.

EMS: So what happens on a day-to-day basis counts less than the movement structure which has been unconsciously choreographed. And what you do is to move or gesture in response to the client's bearing. This, then, is essentially a non-verbal task?

IS: Space and time and energy flow are non-verbal, but they can be expressed verbally. For example, if I ask a client, "What happens to you when I move toward you?" the answer is often a description after the fact. The experiential part of the equation is non-verbal. But I must sense how words are used by the client.

Do they amplify what has been experienced? Often the spoken word is used to ward off or distance from the experience. My work, both in dance and in verbal reflections, must emphasize the opening of the client's space.

EMS: Speaking of space, what kind of facility do you use to do dance therapy?

IS: One defines oneself and needs a place which is conducive to one's professional function. The room that I previously used provided a setting where all the furniture could fold-up and be removed as needed. I currently occupy two sunlit rooms. The smaller of the two serves as the talking room. The back room is very quiet and is multi-purpose and intimate. It is where I do dance therapy.

EMS: So, what I gather, is that your work relates to various formats of movement and arrangement. Spatial and temporal relationships tell the story of relationships, both between you and the client, and the client and the world of others. You've also spoken of boundaries you and the client set. While quite definitive, these boundaries tend toward flexibility and permeability. You appear to focus on the many ways of working with where the client is in functioning in life. And in your understanding, personal rhythm and dance themes define the way you become familiar with the client. The therapeutic processes that you use help the individual move from where he or she is situated to new and more productive places.

IS: Yes, you might sum it up by saying that therapy moves toward emancipation and mutuality. More likely, mutuality becomes the real landmark of the therapeutic process I engage in as a dance therapist.

"To Feel My Own Knowing in Motion": Harmonizing the Mind, Body, and Emotions

Victoria L. Bacon
Barbara L. Fenby
Andrea Mead Lawrence

SUMMARY. The development and meaning of the experience of flow is explored from the perspective of an Olympic athlete. Beginning in childhood and continuing through adolescence, the interaction

Victoria L. Bacon, EdD, is affiliated with the Counseling Program, Bridgewater State College, Bridgewater, MA.

Barbara L. Fenby, DSW, LICSW, is Deputy Area Director, MetroSuburban Area for the Massachusetts Department of Mental Health.

Andrea Mead Lawrence is affiliated with the Mono County Board of Supervisors and is President of the Sierra Nevada Alliance.

Correspondence should be addressed to: Victoria L. Bacon, EdD, Counseling Program, Bridgewater State College, Bridgewater, MA 02325 (E-mail: VBACON@ BRIDGEW.EDU).

[Haworth co-indexing entry note]: " 'To Feel My Own Knowing in Motion': Harmonizing the Mind, Body, and Emotions." Bacon, Victoria L., Barbara L. Fenby, and Andrea Mead Lawrence. Co-published simultaneously in *The Psychotherapy Patient* (The Haworth Press, Inc.) Vol. 10, No. 3/4, 1998, pp. 53-62; and: *Integrating Exercise, Sports, Movement and Mind: Therapeutic Unity* (ed: Kate F. Hays) The Haworth Press, Inc., 1998, pp. 53-62. Single or multiple copies of this article are available for a fee from The Haworth Document Delivery Service [1-800-342-9678, 9:00 a.m. - 5:00 p.m. (EST). E-mail address: getinfo@haworth.com].

53

of instinctual knowing and skill led to flow and culminated in optimal performance–winning a gold medal. Personal narrative within a framework of qualitative research and the professional literature yields an integrated picture of the many facets of flow. *[Article copies available for a fee from The Haworth Document Delivery Service: 1-800-342-9678. E-mail address: getinfo@haworth.com]*

> Mountains are the gift of my birth, not a possession but the bestowal of a natural world where knowledge and this place, my home, unfold together. My parents knew the language of dreams and the words that encourage action, and in the stone castle they built in Vermont and called North Tower, I never knew that dreams and acts are separate for some. (Lawrence & Burnaby, 1980, p. 4)

Through the experience of one of us–Andrea Mead Lawrence, two-time Olympic gold medalist in alpine skiing–we explore the development and meaning of the experience of flow. The narrative excerpts are used to illustrate how, as a young person, Lawrence became aware of the essential elements, which for her led to flow. We then explore how her personally constructed meaning is both unique and similar to the construct of flow found in the literature.

Andrea Mead Lawrence was born in 1932 in Rutland, Vermont and raised at North Tower, her parents' home and a place that remains a symbol of her dreams. Her parents developed and owned a ski area, and with easy access to the slopes, Lawrence learned to ski by the age of five. She skied competitively from 1942-1956, during which time she was a three-time member of the Women's Olympic Alpine Ski Team (1948, 1952, and 1956). In 1952, she won two gold medals, one each in the slalom and giant slalom events. Her later career choices led her to politics, to election to the Mono County Board of Supervisors and to environmental concerns as President of the Sierra Nevada Alliance. Lawrence has five grown children and currently lives in Mammoth Lakes, California.

Lawrence describes her early years as a time when she knew things instinctively, when she felt keenly aware of the natural elements of the outdoors:

> The feeling of the sun on your skin as a child, or the sound of wind, or the color, and the light . . . (Bacon & Fenby, 1995b, p. 18); the sound of the whippoorwills calling . . . (Lawrence & Burnaby, 1980, p. 5); and an absorption which makes me forgetful of myself. (Lawrence, 1996)

Lawrence felt comfortable when alone and very connected with and grounded to the environment. This intimate connection with nature has allowed her to feel at one with the world. Winnicott (1958) suggests that "the capacity to be alone is one of the most important signs of maturity in emotional development" (p. 416). We know that the ability to tolerate being alone is a very difficult task that requires a great deal of concentration, a quality Csikszentmihalyi (1990) has found to be common to persons who report flow-state experiences. Here we see that before the age of ten, Lawrence had experienced a place of centeredness–"physical, mental, emotional equanimity" (Millman, 1994, p. 16).

At the age of ten, Lawrence began skiing competitively. During her first race event she became cognizant of an inner feeling of centeredness, a total conscious awareness and sense of direction with the realization that skiing could give expression to her inner self. She recalls thinking about this awareness as a psychic "click," an inner sense of connection that felt right. Lawrence describes this experience as that of being simultaneously both a spectator and a participant–having an observing ego.

By the age of twelve, Lawrence remembers becoming aware of different personal components of her inner self. Along with the typical identity issues of adolescence, she became acutely aware of having to deal with the physical danger associated with her sport. Ski racing requires a certain amount of courage and daring, given that a racer must negotiate blind spots while racing at high speeds. Racing at Lake Placid, she experienced feelings of fear and apprehension about not being able to see the terrain ahead and about having to deal with uncertainty, the unknown. Instinctively she knew that she had to move through this barrier–her fear and apprehension–which was limiting optimal performance. She struggled to reclaim her earlier self-confidence while having to negotiate her growing awareness of the physical dangers and daring associated with ski racing. Lawrence remembers this as the time when she had to learn to trust what she knew in her mind, having seen and memorized the race course prior to the event. By learning to trust this inner knowing, she was able to race instinctively and again with confidence.

Dealing with fear and apprehension is common among elite athletes. In a recent study on female athletes, competitive and elite athletes viewed fear as a self-motivator. When they were challenged with a fear situation and were able to positively overcome their fear, women reported higher confidence levels that generalized to other areas of their lives (Bacon & Fenby, 1995a). Additionally, it has been suggested that athletes involved in sports where there is danger and sacrifice of comfort often report more startling transcendent experiences (Murphy & White, 1995).

The next level of awareness came for Lawrence at the age of fourteen, after qualifying in New England to go west for the Olympic tryouts in Sun Valley, Idaho. As a youthful competitor she had been a carefree athlete who did not understand the implications of being a member of the Olympic Ski Team. This growing awareness of the internal elements of the athlete is best described by Millman (1994) as developing the "inner athlete." Millman (1994) suggests that enhancing the mental and emotional aspects of the athlete's inner life is as essential as the development of physical skills. He proposes that it is through training that we integrate the body, mind, and emotions (p. xv).

Lawrence was fifteen when she competed in her first Olympics in 1948. As an adolescent she was excited by the experience of traveling by ship to France, then by train to Switzerland, and thus to Olympic competition. But the context of her sporting life had changed dramatically. No longer were training and racing an informal, innocent undertaking. She had a growing conscious awareness of the meaningfulness of competitive skiing and was driven by a sense of responsibility. Lawrence views this time as a transitional period, as she moved from being a naive, energetic racer toward being a world-class ski competitor and an Olympic team member. In this new arena she faced greater external demands and a sense of responsibility for elite performance.

Later that year she was invited to race in the Austrian National Championships, held in Badgastein, which became a very special place for Lawrence. It was here in 1948 that she first became aware of the connection between place and a sense of self which had been with her since childhood in the mountains of Vermont. This connection was and remains very centering.

> At Badgastein in Austria, I never lost a race in all the times I went there, which bespeaks what transpired rather that what I did there. . . . Mountains seem to incline one toward a physics of matter and spirit. They manifest the enormity of nature, which goes beyond division or dualism. The scholastics resolved it by saying that all knowledge lies in the senses. It is a good operating premise when you see life as movement and mountains as symbols. (Lawrence & Burnaby, 1980, p. 20)

Sparked by an inspirational return to her inner association with the mountains and to her past, she went on to win the Austrian National Championships in 1948 and again in Badgastein at other international events in 1951 and 1952.

After winning the National Championships in White Face, Montana in

1949, at the age of sixteen, Lawrence experienced a decline in her ability to perform optimally and did not win any other significant races that year. She remembers that the quality of her racing was very uneven. This period was marked by trial and error with a lot of personal experimentation. Lawrence had no winning runs in this Olympics. In 1950 in Aspen, Colorado during the United States World Championships she recalls trying to ski her best yet experiencing the frustration of not performing well. She felt no sense of inner connectedness and recalls this as a time of internal unrest, a sorting-out of emotions, of feeling pulled in many different directions. Lawrence experienced this as a disappointing year as a competitive racer, a year spent trying to figure out how she had raced when she won the United States Nationals.

Feminist and traditional developmentalists disagree on the nature of female adolescent development, yet they all agree that this period typically involves considerable growth and unrest (Erikson, 1968; Gilligan, 1982; Jordan, Kaplan, Miller, Stiver & Surrey, 1991). Researchers in the field have noted a 25% to 59% attrition rate in the number of female athletes involved in sport between the ages of 11 and 18 (Gould, 1987; Martens, 1978). Several reasons have been suggested, from too much emphasis on competition leading to burnout (Feigley, 1984; Orlick, 1973) to the possibility that young people may take a short break from sport (Gould & Horn, 1984). Further research is needed regarding the implications of gender and sport in our culture. The hope is to lower the drop-out rate of adolescent females, so that they may avail themselves of sports participation.

Nineteen-fifty was a memorable year in that Lawrence got her first full-time coach, Friedle Pfeiffer. Like Lawrence, Pfeiffer had an intuitive sense of skiing; she felt that he made sense. She has always thought of her time with Pfeiffer as her most significant coached experience. Lawrence has come to understand this as a time of intense learning and of great inner growth, which resulted in her movement to another level of maturation. Along with the typical challenges of adolescence, Lawrence was in the process of integrating her "inner athlete." This time must have been incredibly challenging. Optimal performance and flow experience is rooted in a sense of mental, emotional, and physical equilibrium and synthesis, even if momentary. Adolescence, on the other hand, is the very antithesis, a time of emotional upheaval and fragmentation.

Towards the end of 1950, Pfeiffer told Lawrence that he thought that she was burned out and he advised her to stop competing. This suggestion left her feeling devastated. Lawrence recalls feeling shocked—jolted from one level to the next—which served to pull many aspects of herself together. The timing of Pfeiffer's comment served to integrate and solidify the various aspects of her inner life. The evidence of this was clear, for the following week she won the Harriman Cup in downhill, slalom, and combined events in Sun Valley and rarely lost a race after that. Lawrence looks back at this time as progressing from a stage of adolescent immaturity to a more crystallized sense of self. At this time, she moved away from a focus on technique and back to racing instinctively. Her best racing year on a sustained basis was during 1951. It was at this stage that she was able to set a personal goal, to give maximum effort when racing, to put everything on the line.

> I was going to go max out. . . . It was important to do that, and there is an uncompromising quality to that, but more than that was my inner need to extend, to extend myself to the maximum every time I went to the starting gate. . . . I would work on this in my mind, because again, it was something I was evolving and developing. (Bacon & Fenby, 1995b, p. 9)

Lawrence conceptualized her experience as one in which she skied intuitively, having learned to gather, harness, focus, direct, and then release her energy. She became aware that for her these were the essential elements to achieve flow. Lawrence finds the best analogy to describe this process is that of a pressure cooker: a container to gather energy which can be regulated to heighten or release, depending on what is needed. What proved difficult about her conceptualization was that no one in her sport understood this language. Her explanation of how she focused and used her energy was viewed as unique. Although Lawrence had clearly moved into a place of heightened awareness where she was cognizant of the process, this was not easily verbalized nor understood.

> On the plane to Oslo [site of the 1952 Olympics] these many combinations of separate factors governing speed formed again in a larger pattern. The signs set forth came together as a dilated span of personal time without intrusion. . . . I felt its quiet as a reservoir of stillness, without sound and without motion. In skiing I know it as the up of the up, the down of the down; the instant, weightless and lofting, where I pause in the precise middle of momentum. Like the whippoorwills calling through the silence and stillness of summer evenings at North Tower, this reservoir was inclusive. It seemed to summon all that was past, apparently lost in time, and all that remained to be done. (Lawrence & Burnaby, 1980, p. 107)

Lawrence describes her internal process as beginning with the ability to *gather,* to move into a place of stillness. Here she was able to go to the source of her energy–a deep dark pool–a reservoir which was always there. Many things relating to her childhood years–the whippoorwills calling and later the bells ringing in Grindelwald–served as a trigger, to get back to the source, this reservoir. It is from this reservoir that Lawrence was able to *harness* her energy, to be available for action. Next she was able to *focus* on how she would bring all the pieces together. This was done while training on the course to be raced. It was this knowledge about the course together with the reservoir of energy, that would be *directed* to the event and then *released* at the starting gate.

> It's almost as if you have an inner eye and you're seeing the world from a very pure place and you're sort of creating your own sense of direction with it, or it comes from within you somehow, this sense of direction and you see something just with great clarity inside and something in there just keeps moving you that way. (Bacon & Fenby, 1995b, p. 8)

This process of being able to gather, harness, focus, direct, and release was not a physical experience, but a mental, emotional, and spiritual one. This was a defining moment in her life, a time when she put everything that she was and would become on the line. In the first run of the racecourse, Lawrence caught a tip on a gate, spun-off the course and had to quickly climb back up to ski through the missed gate.

> [I]n the first run of the slalom, the odds were against me. . . . The second run of the slalom was my last race in these games. Everything was on the line. One run remained to prove the value of my effort–whether, until now, it had been partial or whole. I had to know if I was real, if the ideal, increasingly refined throughout my career, was possible. (Lawrence & Burnaby, 1980, p. 119)

What Lawrence describes is a moment of altered consciousness, when mind/body/emotions blend, having no awareness of self. This is a moment of complete harmony and it is not until later that the moment is reconstructed by the athlete, and her realness is verified. And so Lawrence's second run of the slalom event at Oslo was indeed her best–a gold medal performance–a defining moment in her life, a transcendent experience (Murphy & White, 1995).

Much of what Lawrence describes is similar to the conceptualization of flow found in psychology and in the sports literature (Csikszentmihalyi, 1988, 1990; Gordin & Reardon, 1995; Jackson, 1995; Leonard, 1990; Millman, 1995; Murphy & White, 1995). Flow can be viewed as the antithesis of dualistic thinking, that Cartesian split in which the body and mind are viewed as separate. Csikszentmihalyi (1990) describes flow as those optimal experiences in which concentration is intense and effortless and where performance and consciousness are harmonious. Lawrence states that for her, we must add the emotional domain. This is consistent with the contention that flow is "a momentary experiential fusing of body, mind, and emotions" (Millman, 1994, p. 110). Although useful to operationally define flow, Leonard (1990), like Murphy and White (1995), reminds us that there are endless possibilities of altered states of consciousness and transcendent experiences in sports. Lawrence's narrative is but one personal account.

The language which Lawrence uses to describe the essential elements and awareness of flow is similar to the hierarchy of skills leading to flow (Gordin & Reardon, 1995). Lawrence describes her process as: gather, harness, focus, direct, and release. In a current text on sport psychology, Gordin and Reardon (1995) categorize the skills necessary for flow as:

1. *Concentration:* the act or process of directing one's attention to a single object;
2. *Composure:* a calmness of mind, body, bearing, and appearance; and
3. *Confidence:* state of mind or consciousness marked by certainty of one's abilities and ease and freedom from doubt (p. 227).

In looking at Lawrence's experience of flow and the ways in which her awareness grew as she progressed developmentally, we have seen that Lawrence holds dear the instinctive knowledge she gained as a young child. She credits the richness of her natural environment, in the mountains of Vermont, as the basis of her instinctive knowing. As an adult Lawrence has come to view instinctive knowing as did the Greek philosophers, Protagoras and Epicurus, or later, Aquinas and William James: all knowledge lies in the senses (DeWulf, 1967; Dooley, 1959; Edwards, 1967; Stodack, 1963). Lawrence contends that the outdoor environment in which she was raised set the stage for her to develop instinctive knowledge via her senses. She believes this provided the foundation for her flow experiences.

Additionally, Lawrence believes that the ability to be alone with oneself is another significant building block in the development of one's emotional sphere. Csikszentmihalyi (1990) suggests that the capacity to be alone is common among athletes who have experienced flow states. These early building blocks allowed Lawrence a calm reservoir to return to when desiring to move into a flow-state experience. As she progressed towards adolescence, Lawrence became aware of having an observing ego. By age twelve she was challenged by the necessary daring and inherent danger associated with ski racing. The decline in optimal performance for Lawrence when she was an adolescent was age appropriate developmentally, as she was in the process of creating her identity. Further, this temporary decline was partially a result of her intense attention to technique development. And lastly, we see that she experienced internal integration and was then able to call upon the essential elements to achieve flow.

This has been Lawrence's subjective narrative. She constructed her own personal epistemology or way of knowing (Belenky, Clinchy, Goldberger, & Tarule, 1986), in which she developed and gave personal meaning to her experience of flow. Viewed in a stage progression of increased awareness of the essential elements of flow, we have considered how Lawrence moved from a fun-loving, intuitive youngster to an adolescent with a more crystallized sense of self and then to a world-class athlete. Lawrence's narrative excerpts demonstrate that her ability to conceptualize and her ability to perform are related. In Lawrence's words, to perform is "to feel my own knowing in motion" (Lawrence & Burnaby, 1980, p. 35).

REFERENCES

Bacon, V.L. & Fenby, B.L. (1995a). The identity of the female athlete. *Massachusetts Psychological Quarterly, 39*(3), 4.

Bacon, V.L. & Fenby, B.L. (1995b). [Research narratives of female athletes across the lifespan.] Unpublished raw data.

Belenky, M.F., Clinchy, B.M., Goldberger, N.R. & Tarule, J.M. (1986). *Women's ways of knowing: The development of self, voice, and mind.* NY: Basic Books, Incorporated.

Csikszentmihalyi, M. (1988). *Optimal experience: Psychological studies of flow in consciousness.* NY: Cambridge University Press.

Csikszentmihalyi, M. (1990). *Flow.* NY: Harper Perennial.

DeWulf, M. (1959). *The system of Thomas Aquinas.* NY: Dover Publishers Incorporated.

Dooley, P.K. (1974). *Pragmatism as humanism: The philosophy of William James.* Chicago: Nelson-Hall.

Edwards, P. (1967). *The encyclopedia of philosophy,* Vol. 7 (pp. 415-419). NY: The Macmillan Company & The Free Press.

Erikson, E. (1968). *Identity: Youth and crisis.* NY: W.W. Norton.

Feigley, D.A. (1984). Psychological burnout in high-level athletes. *The Physician and Sports Medicine, 12*(10), 108-119.

Gilligan, C. (1982). *In a different voice.* Cambridge, MA: Harvard University Press.

Gordin R.D. & Reardon, J.P. (1995). Achieving the zone: The study of flow in sport. In K.P. Henschen and W.F. Straub (Eds). *Sport psychology as analysis of athlete behavior* (3rd ed.) Ann Arbor: Mouvement Publications.

Gould, D. (1987). Understanding attrition in children's sports. In D. Gould & M.R. Weiss (Eds.). *Advances in pediatric sport sciences,* Vol. 2, Behavioral Issues (pp. 61-85). Champaign, IL: Human Kinetics.

Gould, D. & Horn, T. (1984). Participation motivation in young athletes. In J.M. Silva & R.S. Weinberg (Eds.), *Psychological foundations of sport* (pp. 359-370). Champaign, IL: Human Kinetics.

Jackson, S. (1995). Factors influencing the occurrence of flow state in elite athletes. *Journal of Applied Sport Psychology, 7*, 138-166.

Jordan, J.V., Kaplan, A.G., Miller, J.B., Stiver, I.P. & Surrey, J.L. (1991). *Women's growth in connection.* NY: Guilford Press.

Lawrence, A.M. (1996). Personal communication.

Lawrence, A.M. & Burnaby, S. (1980). *A Practice of mountains.* NY: Seaview Books.

Leonard, G. (1990). *The ultimate athlete.* Berkeley, CA: North Atlantic Books.

Martens, R. (1978). *Joy and sadness in children's sport.* Champaign, IL: Human Kinetics.

Millman, D. (1994). *The inner athlete.* Walpole, NH: Stillpoint Publishing.

Murphy, M. & White, R.A. (1995). *In the zone.* NY: Penguin Books.

Orlick, T.D. (1973, January/February). Children's sport—A revolution is coming. *Canadian Association for Health Physical Education and Recreation Journal,* 21-27.

Strodach, G.K. (1963). *The philosophy of Epicurus.* Northwestern University Press.

Winnicott, D.W. (1958). The capacity to be alone. *The International Journal of Psychoanalysis, 39*, 416-420.

Relational Aspects of Competition:
A Father Learns from His Daughters

Timothy J. Wildman

SUMMARY. Utilizing the dual contexts of feminist relational psychology and the writer's acculturation to sport as a male, his daughters' competitive running relationships are explored. With the 1995 Boston Marathon as a central unifying event and metaphor, it is concluded that: relatedness and competitiveness are an empowering tension; men feel a need to bifurcate relatedness and competitiveness; and a sport such as running can foster relational growth. Girls and women, entering competitive sports in ever-increasing numbers, should be encouraged to retain and develop their relational skills in order to achieve maximum performance and attain optimal benefit. The infusion of relational values can increase the enjoyment of competitive sport by both females and males. *[Article copies available for a fee from The Haworth Document Delivery Service: 1-800-342-9678. E-mail address: getinfo@haworth.com]*

The 6:00 a.m. New Hampshire air is biting but the April sun lies before us like a promise as my daughters, my wife, and I pile into the car. It is April 15, 1995, and the women in my life and I are heading south pursuing a first marathon for my 23-year-old daughter, Abby, and me. My younger daughter, Rachel, and my wife, Carol, are the support troops. In the car, laughter and teasing mix with tension and unease.

While I have run since 1980 (mostly for stress reduction and enjoy-

Timothy J. Wildman, DMin, is affiliated with Cornerstone Family Resources, Concord, NH.

[Haworth co-indexing entry note]: "Relational Aspects of Competition: A Father Learns from His Daughters." Wildman, Timothy J. Co-published simultaneously in *The Psychotherapy Patient* (The Haworth Press, Inc.) Vol. 10, No. 3/4, 1998, pp. 63-80; and: *Integrating Exercise, Sports, Movement and Mind: Therapeutic Unity* (ed: Kate F. Hays) The Haworth Press, Inc., 1998, pp. 63-80. Single or multiple copies of this article are available for a fee from The Haworth Document Delivery Service [1-800-342-9678, 9:00 a.m. - 5:00 p.m. (EST). E-mail address: getinfo@haworth.com].

ment), I had long since given up the idea of running a marathon. "Too much time for training," I had told myself. But Abby, who was working in Boston after college, had seen her first Boston Marathon in '94, come home, and called me: "Dad, we've gotta do it–you know we do!" And here we were–on our way to the 99th running of Boston, prepared to take our places with the other "Back of the Pack Gang," runners described as "bandits" because we were "stealing" our way into the race as unregistered runners.

I began running because a neighbor talked me into it. I had run on my own a few times through the years but had never stuck with it. When my neighbor said that he was looking for someone to go with him, I told him I would give it a try. Later that summer we were joined by a third friend. Within the next two years, my neighbor moved away, but the third friend has run with me since, and we have forged a relationship characterized by its own kind of intimacy through the years.

"Intimacy" is also the very word that describes the kind of relationship developed between my daughters and me via our running for the past few years. The quality of our "run talks" usually surpasses conversations held at the dinner table, on the phone, or even in the car. Closeness, honesty, and mutuality have prevailed. In this atmosphere I've learned a lot, not only about them but also about the "relational" way in which they approach running and competition.

I have been greatly assisted in understanding this relational view by the "Self-in-Relation" perspective of women's psychological development offered by theorists associated with the Stone Center at Wellesley College. Surrey, for example, comments, "for women, the primary experience of self is relational, that is, the self is organized and developed in the context of important relationship" (1991b, p. 52). This model is contrasted with the traditional separation/individuation model of development. These theorists feel the traditional model does not accurately describe women's "process of growth within relationships, where both or all people involved are encouraged and challenged to maintain connection and to foster, adapt to, and change with the growth of the other" (Surrey, 1991b, p. 60). For my daughters, late adolescence has been a key period for the formation of women's "core relational self structure." The "complexity, flexibility, sensitivity, and adaptability" of this self structure increase dramatically during this period, laying out the pathways for the future (Gleason, Kaplan, & Klein, 1991).

My daughters have been in college during this period and their experience echoes the perspective of Belenky, Clinchy, Goldberger, and Tarule (1986) that women in the educational process know things differently than the dominant male culture may understand. "Connected knowing" describes my daughters' inclinations to learn through utilizing their own subjectivity and experience as well as through what they are taught by others. "Constructed knowing" elucidates their emerging sense of knowing in the dynamic interaction between "knower and known." The remarkable vitality of my daughters' "run talk" both about running and about other aspects of their lives has the quality of what these authors refer to as the "real talk of the constructivist" (Belenky et al., 1986, p. 144).

Carol Gilligan (1989) eloquently describes the "underground world" with "caverns of knowledge" which extensive conversations with adolescent girls reveal. She expresses the dilemma of voicelessness in girls and women, as well as the moral conflict inherent in being asked by the culture to give up the self in order to maintain connection to the culture. I see these dilemmas and conflicts in my daughters' lives and have found running to be a forum for my increased understanding.

The interrelation of gender, relationship, and sport can be understood from a sports perspective as well. Hill and Oglesby (1995) advocate for a specific balance. Traditional male sporting values include independence, activity, ruled and bounded behavior, and the opponent as the challenge. "Transformed sport" values provide further enrichment through balancing these traditional values with dependence/interdependence, passivity/quiet, chaotic/inventive/improvisation, and love/care for the challenger.

MY OWN HISTORY OF RELATIONAL DYNAMICS AND COMPETITION

What follows is a brief history of the relational dynamics in my development and the view of competition with which I grew up. As a young boy, I felt different from others, more drawn to what I would now call the relational aspects of life than my male peers. I was not in any way naturally gifted in sports. I did, however, have a passion for them from as early as I can remember, in large part stimulated by my only sibling, a brother who was 6 years older. He patiently taught me both the rules and techniques of basketball, baseball and eventually football. Even though he played few of these sports himself beyond the age of 14, I was always in awe of his natural abilities as an athlete and as my teacher. While I had typical boyhood fantasies of being the lone sports hero, like Mickey Mantle hitting the ninth-inning homerun or Otto Graham tossing the winning touchdown pass, what I seemed to like most about sports was being part of a team or part of the social experience of playing the game. I was always the one who called everyone until I could get enough boys together for a sandlot baseball game. In order to tempt my friends to stop for a game of one-on-one basketball on their way home from school, I shoveled the snow off the basketball court in winter. I loved practice and did quite well when the outcome "didn't matter." On the other hand, I detested games. The zenith of my career in team sports came in my senior year in high school when I was the sixth man on a basketball team that won 1 and lost 18. My coach during these years (a true "screamer") was frequently successful in shaming me. The bulging veins on his neck made it clear to me that I lacked both skill and natural aggression. His most common advice regarding my poor performance in games was that I was insufficiently able to "get mad."

My coach might similarly critique the only sport which I have carried forward from adolescence: tennis. I have what might best be described as a love/hate relationship with this sport. In tennis, one must face one's opponent directly across a net. On that rare occasion when I might be winning and my opponent becomes frustrated with himself, I am immediately drawn to his distress. As I am increasingly drawn to this distress, I lose focus on my own game and become swept away in a rapidly turning tide of athletic codependency. My opponent wins again. Being so drawn to the pain of the competitor that I feel it necessary to sacrifice my own winning in order to enable my opponent's happiness would drive my coach crazy. But from a relational perspective it fits me somehow.

All these early relational inclinations and my subsequent experiences in sports should make me a male who could understand and relate well to his daughters and their competitive endeavors. This has not necessarily been true, however. Despite my sense of relatedness, as a male socialized in this culture core beliefs about competition are embedded in my psyche:

1. Performance and achievement are the goals of sport; relationships are a by-product. They are nice but not essential and may be irrelevant or needlessly cumbersome.
2. Heroism is individual.
3. Effective leadership is hierarchical.
4. Your opponent is an enemy to be defeated or even annihilated. Thus, aggression is necessary. Nice guys finish last.

Janet Surrey articulates the prevalent notion inherent in my "truths": "relationships are something you have when you are not working or living your life" (1991a, p. 162). In the last few years, I have been surprised at how much my experience with my daughters has been determined by these core beliefs. For this reason their relational values about sport and competition were not well understood by me at first. Gradually, with much interest and some humility, my consciousness of these relational values has been raised.

RELATEDNESS AND COMPETITIVENESS: AN EMPOWERING TENSION

It is now mid-morning. After parking the car we are all bused to the sun-drenched center of little Hopkinton, Massachusetts. The temperature is now in the mid-forties. We begin stretching as an alternative to pacing. From amidst the meandering throng of runners and spectators, Rachel's college friend, Sarah, emerges with her boyfriend. She, too, is marathon-bound in the bandit lane.

Rachel met Sarah early in their freshman year of college. Before the year was through, Sarah had come home with Rachel and spent a week with us. Each girl had experienced their parents' divorce in the previous few years. They were united in spirit by a shared sense of the familial decimation and interpersonal frustration that divorces almost always produce. In other ways, however, they were different. My daughter is serious about her studies and worries constantly about her academic performance. Although Sarah has virtually had to finance her own education and values it greatly, she is also spontaneous and teaches Rachel how to have fun.

Like Rachel, Sarah is an athlete, having arrived on campus as a soccer player. Last year, on what began as a lark, Sarah started to run more seriously, eventually defeating Rachel in a summer road race. In talks with her friends and me, Rachel was able to articulate her sense of betrayal in response to her friend's interest and performance level in the sport of my daughter's choosing. Her ambivalent feelings toward her friend troubled her. She cared deeply for her and felt close to her, yet she felt threatened by being eclipsed in her own field. The competitiveness and relatedness, while not strained to the breaking point, coexisted in an uneasy peace. This competitive/relational tension did not separate them, however. Gleason, Kaplan, and Klein observe that "the intense affective quality with which conflict is expressed can represent a means by which young women work out differences within relationships, moving into a relationship to confront differences, not away from it" (1991, p. 125).

Amidst this tension Rachel and Sarah (who were to room together again) agreed to go forward as cross-country teammates in the fall if Sarah didn't make the starting soccer team when they returned to school. Two weeks into the school year, they became teammates as well as roommates. In most of the races, Rachel, who races in the first position and is the co-captain, has prevailed over her friend. But in at least one or two, she has lost to Sarah. In competitive fields numbering as many as 300 young women they usually finish in sequential order, and the difference in their times is only a few seconds. After these races Rachel calls home and expresses her feelings of ambivalence, especially if she has lost to her friend. When I have been present for a race, however, I've observed that within only a few minutes of the end of the race, the two have become able to acknowledge and share their competitive feelings (usually with humor), their joy in their performances, and their plans to do even better in the next race. That their relationship is enhancing each person's performance is undeniable. What is more stunning to me is that two women still so young in their own development can work through, week by week, their very real feelings of competitiveness within the context of relatedness without feeling it necessary to silence the competitiveness or break the relatedness.

In one of her post-race calls, Rachel recalled that she and Sarah had run together as far into the race as they could, pushing the pace for each other. When one could no longer keep pace, they continued to periodically yell each other's name to "stay in touch" until the race's conclusion—a real-life illustration of Surrey's definition of relationships as "the ongoing, intrinsic inner awareness and responsiveness to the continuous existence of the other or others and the expectation of mutuality in this regard" (1991b, p. 61).

Such mutually responsive relationships between and among members of the same sports team have traditionally been called "teamwork." Even professional athletes talk more about teamwork in post-game television interviews than about individual performance. Thus, this old value would seem to be alive and well. A darker side to sport, however, is revealed by the attention, money, and value bestowed upon the individual heroism and performance of athletes. Trash talk and other forms of one-on-one opponent-baiting get at least as much air time as teamwork. Perhaps it will be from women that the world of sports is reminded about the performance-enhancing aspects of teamwork. A sports team could, in this context, be seen as "the new relational unit . . . (which) comes to have a unique existence beyond the individuals, to be attended to, cared about, and nurtured . . . (where) the self gains vitality and enhancement in relationships and is not reduced or threatened by connections" (Surrey, 1991b, p. 62). The interaction between Sarah and Rachel inspires my hope that this may happen.

My optimism about an infusion of relational values in sports is bolstered in a different way by the following story. Earlier this year, I had the privilege of witnessing my daughter win a fairly large Division III cross-country invitational. The race, run on a dank and rainy day, featured an exciting finish in which Rachel overtook her mud-covered opponent by a step at the finish line. She later told me that only the week before she had beaten the same young woman near the end of the race. On the occasion of this second close loss the competitor said to Rachel, "Did you know I was trying to work with you during the race?" My daughter immediately understood that her opponent had been reaching out to her to create the kind of connection from which they could play off each other's energy to enhance both their performances. Upon hearing this, my daughter embraced her, thanked her, and added teasingly that in the next race she would know that any elbows she got in the ribs were only part of "working together." Rachel did not relate this story with any surprise, but I was mystified that two competitors working so hard to defeat each other could also be working together. These two young women rather dramatically overcame what Gilligan names as the dilemma of teenage girls and adult women: "(is) it better to respond to others and abandon themselves or to respond to themselves and abandon others?" (1989, p. 9). Hill and Ogelesby's "transformed sport" model provides a way to conceptualize this balancing of self and other. The competitive endeavor involves love/care for the challenger.

Rachel and her opponent were competing with each other–relationally. Such relational competition has traditionally been referred to as "sportsmanship." If teamwork involves relatedness to teammates, sportsmanship involves relatedness to opponents. In a recent rare occurrence in a World Series, a brush-back pitch emptied both benches in a brawl. While the vast majority of players from both teams either fought with each other or pulled their teammates off one another, the two pitchers stood out by the pitcher's mound and chatted. During a post-game interview, one of the pitchers commented that having the opportunity in the midst of a game to talk with the opposing pitcher had been a rare and wonderful opportunity. As I reflected on this event, it was not only the pitchers' relating to each other that was remarkable, it was also their ability to understand its significance that was unusual. Right there on television, two models for contending were being presented: brawling and talking. Of course, some of what was going on in the talking was mental competition. Conversely, some of those who were brawling were not doing so with true conviction but rather with a kind of obligatory resignation. Nevertheless, as behavioral alternatives, brawling and talking offer stark contrast. Unfortunately, the talking pitchers are rare in contemporary male sport. Again, relational values are needed in order to remind the culture of sport about the value of sportsmanship and the ways in which sportsmanship can enhance performance.

A FATHER LEARNS ABOUT RUNNING AND RELATEDNESS

As "the hour" approaches, Abby and I complete what has now become nearly simultaneous hydration and elimination, say goodbye to Rachel and Carol who are to meet us at Mile 18 (Heartbreak Hill), and ease our way into the back of the pack like uncertain bathers wading into a roiling ocean. Now it is just the two of us. On a shared training run several weeks earlier, I told Abby that I would have completed a milestone in my life and relationship with her not when we crossed the finish line but when we toed the start line. That moment has arrived.

When my children were young, I had typical father fantasies about the heroic sports achievements my children might one day attain. Abby, my oldest child, showed little interest in sports until seventh grade when she decided to try running the mile for the track team. I still remember her returning from her runs around the neighborhood red-faced and out of breath. After a time, she allowed me to run with her on occasion. While I spent the entire time trying to coach her on how she might view the psychology of racing and conditioning (subjects about which I knew little or nothing), my internal experience was that I simply enjoyed running and being with her in that way.

After this brief flirtation with running, Abby went back to a life without sports. She occasionally came home humorously describing misadventures in required gym class but had little interest in sports beyond this. She always followed her sister's athletic endeavors with interest and support but never seemed able to relate to this in any personal way. However, during the spring term of her junior year in college, which she spent in Russia, she found that a combination of factors of life in the deteriorating USSR of 1992 and her own personal trials led to a level of stress that worried her. Somehow, out of this matrix of factors, she came to feel that running would be the best way to reduce this stress. She learned almost immediately that it suited her. During a lay-over in Finland on her way home from Russia she ran in a forest outside of Helsinki and found it to be one of the most thrilling experiences of her life. When she returned home, she did little running over the summer but in her senior year began to run regularly for stress reduction and recreation. A young woman at her student job convinced Abby to join her in training for a half-marathon in early May of that year. Phone calls home increasingly made reference to her runs and their distance. A new element began to surface as well–time. She refused to buy a runner's watch to keep exact time, but I could hear that the approximate times of her runs were becoming more important to her as the possibility of actually completing the race became more real. She decided to enter a 7-mile race the week before the half-marathon and asked me to come. I packed up my 9-month-old son, Tyler, and went off to an exciting and heart-warming day in which he and I saw Abby run her first-ever race in the morning and Rachel run her best time yet in a 2-miler that afternoon in the same town. While I was delighted with each of their performances, it was not clear to me at the time how much Abby was seeking to deepen and enhance our relationship through her interest in running.

This reaching out came at a time in my daughter's development when traditional separation/individuation theories would anticipate "breaking away" as the central developmental theme. Within a relational framework, Stern (1990) notes that young adolescent girls experience both separation and connection. As girls grow older and more independent, "others can be appreciated as people rather than as instrumental providers," and "relationships (then) provide the support one needs to push one's own development further" (Stern, p. 84). In our "running relationship" Abby looked for some of the relational vitality she needed to be who she was becoming.

One year after Abby had run her first race, she asked me to join her in the same 7-miler, a beautiful loop around one end of a lake in New Hampshire. Carol, Tyler, Rachel, Abby and I all piled into the car to make a day of it. The race was always followed by a hearty cookout and a keg of beer. Abby had now graduated and was living in Boston. She had matured remarkably during that time, with an increasingly well-developed view of herself and the world. As we warmed up for the race, I was aware of my respect for her as a person and my fondness for her as a friend as well as a daughter. With high hopes of a good time together, we began the race at the sound of the gun.

If Abby and I were to run together I knew that I would need to slow my race pace. On the other hand, I knew that my daughter had been training and would probably run at a good pace for her. In a way that was reminiscent of our runs when she was in the seventh grade, I began to offer advice about how we needed to deal with race strategy (something about which I now knew not a great deal more than I had 10 years earlier). My daughter seemed reluctant to give herself over to what I regarded as the competitive fun of the race, so after the first mile, we talked and kidded, enjoyably passing the time together. We finished in a pace just over 8-minute miles, a respectable time for me and an excellent time for her.

When we were joined by the rest of the family following the race, I was taken aback by my daughter's description of my behavior during the race. "Dad spent the entire race wanting to pass people. All he wanted to do was pass people, pass people. He was especially bad about women, 'we've gotta pass that woman up there.' I couldn't believe it! What's that about,

Dad?" I tried to explain to her that I was only concerned about passing women so that her place in the women's race would be improved. She seemed skeptical if not downright disbelieving. What I had considered to be the competitive fun of the race she saw as an inability to simply be present in the race experience and enjoy it. I kidded her that all she wanted to do was "meet people and talk like this was some sort of social event." Her response: "So what's so bad about that?"

Once again, I had felt that competing was the defining factor in the race. From my perspective, this would mean passing as many people as possible and being aware of your own numerical standing in your race group. While not completely unimportant to Abby, this element of the race was inseparable from our relatedness to each other and the relatedness which she felt to other people that she might meet in the race or whom she might already know. This race marked the beginning of a running relatedness between us that would eventually carry us to a marathon.

In the earlier years of our running, my friend and I had fantasized about running a marathon. For several years we trained for and ran a 12.5-mile race and wondered with awe about what it might be like to run a distance more than twice that far. As the years passed, however, our responsibilities as parents and spouses and increasing career demands made our fantasy an ever-dimming vision. Just a few years ago I told my friend I had finally let go of the fantasy altogether and was happy to run for conditioning and an occasional race. Thus, I was startled to notice how quickly I signed on to Abby's proposal that we run the Boston Marathon together. From the beginning she had great confidence that this was something we could accomplish. We were both aware that to run Boston you must qualify with another marathon at a fairly fast pace. I *was* able to be emphatic that I was *not* going to run two marathons. It would be a miracle if I could run one! So from the beginning, we resolved to run with several thousand other unregistered runners in the "back of the pack gang."

Throughout the year before the marathon, we talked weekly on the phone about our mileage and training efforts. I never ran more than 4 times a week, as I felt my aging body would not tolerate more than this. Abby, on the other hand, ran almost every day and cross trained in the small gym at the hospital where she worked. When she was home for a weekend or a holiday, we ran together, often choosing these occasions for our long runs. Four months before the marathon, we began our training in earnest, running the long miles through the New England winter and interspersing our runs with phone calls characterized by increasingly warm, funny, and knowledgeable talk about our preparation. My daughter gave me a marathon training book for Christmas. We took some of its advice where helpful, but we also vowed not to "get compulsive about this." We were certainly not compulsive, but we were increasingly committed.

MEN AND THE DISAVOWAL OF RELATEDNESS OR COMPETITIVENESS

A "frat party" atmosphere prevails among us non-registered types with a preponderance of college kids and people in funny headgear and outfits. News helicopters hover above as palpable waves of excitement undulate across the crowd and ripple through my GI tract. It takes us 11 minutes after the gun sounds to reach the start line and another 2 or 3 minutes to start intermittent jogging. But at least we are finally moving!

Abby and I agree that we will check the clock at each early mile to keep a pace of 9-minute miles or slower, as we both fear burning out and not finishing. We also decide that we will run this race together. Whatever happens to one happens to both.

The early miles are exciting and seem to go by effortlessly and quickly. The crowds for the Boston Marathon are legendary for being supportive and enthusiastic. This year is no exception. Abby is wearing a college sweatshirt and all along the way people cheer her on with "Go, Dartmouth!" She tells me that I am included in this cheer as well, since I paid for much of the Dartmouth education—a generous offer which I accept.

In Natick, a little after Mile 10, we come upon two men in their 50s discussing their ultra-marathoning (50 or 100 mile races) exploits in the same tone that intellectuals might analyze Proust or determinism in a coffee house. Abby chuckles at the "maleness" of their oneups-manship.

On one of her mid-winter morning training runs Abby passed two men in their sixties several hundred yards apart. Near the end of her run, she came upon the two of them again. This time they were walking together and hailed her. They asked if she was a member of the local running club, and she responded that she didn't even know that running clubs existed. They were incredulous but proceeded to give her some information about the value of such a club. Wanting to be conversational, she asked them how many years they had been running together. They immediately responded with one voice that they did *not* run together. They ran separately—as fast as they could. They had been coming out here for over 20 years at the same time each morning (in what amounted to a daily foot race) and often ended up walking together at the end of their route to cool down. They were emphatic that this did not constitute "running together."

Abby found this hilarious. We both saw that their relationship with each other was a significant part of what had given meaning to their performance through the years. Yet they found it necessary to deny this related-ness while simultaneously benefiting from it. Surrey's observation that "men do not have as many opportunities for developing their relational capacities and do not learn to develop trust in their capacity to engage in mutually empathic, mutually empowering interaction" (1991a, p.168) sets an interesting context for the early morning "races" of these two tradi-tional males.

My running partner and I have, over the many years, evolved a more subtle strategy for managing competitiveness and relatedness. For 10 years or more we ran the same 7.5-mile course three mornings a week. Throughout the route we pushed each other, taking turns with pacing. We never acknowledged this, however, saying instead that we were only keep-ing up with the other. In this way, we managed to deny any competitive-ness while remaining related. This strategy emerged without discussion. From the very beginning, however, one segment of the route, a steep uphill section between Miles 5 and 6, was silently declared off-limits to our relational connection. During this stretch, we each had unspoken permis-sion to go as fast as we could–in a way, it was a race. Invariably one of us would arrive at the top first and run in place until the other arrived. We then finished the last mile-and-a-half together. Being somewhat younger than the two males in Abby's story, my friend and I were perhaps genera-tionally able to preserve the relatedness of our running. We both acknowl-edged that this relatedness was the most important reason we ran at all. Interestingly, what we denied was our competitiveness. The lesson for males here, complicated and convoluted though it may be, is that relation-ships can enhance competitiveness and competitiveness can strengthen relationships.

BUILDING AND MAINTAINING RELATEDNESS THROUGH SPORTS

I am keeping track of our pace mile by mile. At Mile 16 Abby asks how we've done the last mile. I respond "it doesn't matter now—we just have to focus on finishing." I'm shifting from coaching to surviving. Abby's energy also begins to wane, and she develops some breathing difficulties. She occasionally has asthmatic problems and has not brought her inhaler with her. As we get into the Hills section, she finds running even more labored but continues, with my encouragement, to go forward. It seems that as one of us feels, so both of us feel.

We see Carol and Rachel on Heartbreak Hill, and I worry that Abby will be discouraged as we learn that her inhaler is not available. She takes on water and some Gatorade, however, and literally seems to get a "second wind." Rachel joins us at this point, and the three of us ascend the last mile of Heartbreak Hill together. As I have been warned, we now hit the infamous marathon "wall" and begin the most difficult portion of the race on the descent into Boston. I become wooden-legged and overwhelmingly fatigued. I think "I just want to lie down over by the curb and go to sleep." I can no longer keep up with what is now Abby's 9.5-minute-per-mile pace, and ruefully remember my earlier fantasies of running a marathon in under 8-minute miles. Abby is running 15, then 25, yards ahead of me. Rachel runs back and forth between the two of us, coming back for seemingly casual conversation. In fact, I later learn she is taking scouting reports back to her older sister. The middle of my three older children, Rachel now enacts literally and symbolically what she does best—bridging and reaching out.

It became apparent early in my second child's life that she would probably be the most athletically gifted member of our family. From an early age, she was interested in soccer, softball and basketball. My third child, Matthew, never liked sports. He tried them, doubtless out of respect for me. But by the age of 9 or 10 he had made it clear that "I'm never gonna do anything where I have to sweat." Thus, from the time of Rachel's grade school days, I could see that it would be primarily with her that I would share my love of sports.

The children's mother and I separated and divorced when Rachel was an eighth grader. That year, she played soccer and softball. From this point forward, attending her sporting events became the most consistent opportunity for us to relate through some rocky times in our relationship. An essay she wrote as a senior in high school revealed that she had always understood the role sports played in our relationship: "I was the only child in my family who played sports and enjoyed it. It was the one thing that drew me and my father closer." It was this already-established relational link which supported us through the difficult years of her adolescence—a link she understood long before I did. I am only now beginning to appreciate the relational complexity which our shared interest in sports has supported, a complexity which she grasped and modulated with a great deal more sophistication than I.

Rachel had great passion for sports but felt she achieved only modest success through grammar school and junior high. Her sophomore year in high school, however, one of her friends convinced her to go out for track, and a previously undiscovered part of her began to emerge. As she commenced training and then racing with increasing competitive success, I could see that she was developing a different kind of confidence in her abilities generally. The father in me experienced some relief that she was finally beginning to "get it" about the importance of competing and winning. In only her second year of running, she qualified for the league championship meet in the 800 meters. She was apprehensive about this and talked to me at some length about it (one of the few things about which she was talking to me at that point). I was thrilled–that she had qualified for this level of competition *and* that she was talking to me. I was proud of her and told her so repeatedly. When I talked to her a half hour before her race, she expressed some concern for her best friend who had qualified in the same heat. Her friend was experiencing some mild stomach cramps and wasn't sure she would be able to run. In my competitive male way, I encouraged my daughter to focus on her own performance and not be sidetracked by other matters. She listened silently and told me she needed to warm up.

The 800-meter race is only two laps long. It was therefore with something that retrospectively I can only describe as horror that I observed Rachel running the entire first lap looking over her shoulder. At the end of the first lap, she seemed to wake up and begin running in earnest. By then it was too late, and she finished with an unusually poor time. I tried to be as patient and affirming after the race as possible. She was clearly disappointed in herself and her performance, but when I asked her why she had been looking over her shoulder, she stared at me as if the reason should have been obvious: "Well didn't you know that I was on the outside and Erica was in the far inside lane and I couldn't see her. That whole first lap I couldn't see her; I didn't know if she was still running, or had dropped out, or if she was even okay. By the time I knew that she was still running, it was too late." In the discussion that followed, I continued to try to be patient, listen well, and understand her behavior.

What I didn't fully comprehend then but can see now was that for her, relationship with her friend and competition were inseparable. She truly regretted her sub-par performance, but she would not have acted differently had the same circumstances occurred again. What I initially saw as an inability to focus on the task at hand (or worse, as a whimsical and immature interest in a friendship at a moment where such an interest was unnecessary), I now see as part of the fabric of relatedness that is woven through my daughter's experience of competition and through her sports relationship with me.

RELATEDNESS AND EMPOWERMENT

As I have learned more from Rachel about maintaining relatedness through sports, I have also begun to understand how her sports relationships can be mutually empowering. Her way of captaining her college cross country team emphasizes this mutual empowerment. At its best, the role of being a captain on a sports team is always a relational one. Captaining is ideally characterized by an interdependent mode of leadership in which "each person contributes equally and the importance of the individual's involvement is judged in terms not only of contributions but also of the involvement of each member" (Hanmer, Lyons, and Saltonstall, 1990, p. 207). This interdependent leadership includes modeling self-discipline and dedication as highly valued aspects of team involvement. Further, the captains' involved interaction with team members enables greater levels of endeavor and performance.

Rachel's way of captaining her team with her co-captain cohorts, however, is done at a relational level well beyond what I had experienced on team sports myself. She seems highly aware of her relationships: with the coach and her wishes for the team, with her co-captain colleagues, and with the team members. She likes chatting on the phone every evening with her charges about that day's training regimen or the stress of school (fitting athletic performance into an academically rigorous Division III school). She especially enjoys captaining the freshmen, some of whom have done only minimal competitive running before joining the team in college. She describes activities designed to build morale and deepen the enjoyment for all members of the team: pasta dinners prepared by the captains for the men's and women's teams combined, gelatin-square-making parties for energy food on the night before races, and special hikes.

Other team members, the coach, and parents talk at races about the atmosphere of fun, relaxation and close relationship created by the coach and her captains. In this environment many of the less experienced runners are obviously performing well beyond their own or others' expectations. Rachel seems confident that people can be motivated to go beyond such thresholds through trust in consistent and meaningful relationships. The team's experience this year embodies the concept of "power with others, that is, power in connection or relational power. Thus we have talked about mutual empowerment (each person is empowered) through relational empowerment (the relationship is empowered)" (Surrey, 1991a, p. 163). In sports we might add: the team is empowered.

CONCLUSION

My "go-between" daughter is now trying to captain her father—ever more directively. She advises: "Pick up your knees or your feet will trip you!" At the final water stop a couple of miles before the finish line, I walk for 15 or 20 steps, as is our custom at each water stop. I have barely begun running again when I quickly decide that walking felt better. Rachel again takes me in hand: "If you don't start running within the next 20 feet, you'll never run again!" The last two miles seem endless, but when we turn the corner for what Rachel informs me are the final 400 meters on Boylston Street, life seems to come into my body from somewhere and we sprint down the final sun-filled stretch—a daughter on each side and a father in the middle.

Crossing the finish line is a golden moment. We have finished in a time of 4 hours and 10 minutes. More to the point, we have finished—together.

I lean on Abby and Rachel, refuse an offer to go into the medical tent, and eventually meet up with Carol to whom my first words are: "I'm never doing this again." A chronic marathoner tells me I will change my mind, but I haven't. I don't need to do another marathon. The achievement is not about running 26 miles; it is about spending a remarkable year in my life planning and preparing for it with one daughter and then having an experience with both daughters which is almost indescribable in its joy and depth. The marathon undertaking I had considered virtually impossible a few years before is now indelibly linked to my relationships with these daughters. I now truly believe that relationships can empower one to accomplish things previously felt to be impossible. I also believe that my daughters had always known this.

Every year many of the self-in-relation theorists gather for a conference entitled "Learning From Women." When I attended this gathering, and listened as a relational way of viewing psychology and life in general emerged from the presentations, I felt taught and inspired. As I left the conference I found myself musing that so many areas of life and culture needed to "learn from women": global politics, religion, economics, and ecology just to name a few. The lessons learned from my daughters lead me to add "sports" to this list.

Yet learning from women in the field of sports will not occur easily. As I described the subject matter of this article to some friends who are mothers of school-age female athletes, they observed that in fact their daughters were learning the intense, cut-throat, male style of competition from mostly male coaches. They were skeptical that girls and women would bring relational values to sports, but felt instead that (once again) females would learn to adapt to male values in a predominantly male sports-world. I hope they are wrong, for the world of sports and competition greatly needs an infusion of relatedness. The empowering tension between relatedness and competitiveness, the performance value of relatedness, the ways in which relatedness can be maintained through sports, and the remarkable manner in which relatedness empowers athletes to do that which seemed unlikely or even impossible, are all elements of such an infusion.

For this infusion to have a chance of success, the relational inclinations of girls and young women in sports must be encouraged rather than submerged beneath male ideas of competition. My own male inclination to dismiss, minimize, misunderstand, try to correct, or downright ignore these relational inclinations in my daughters is sad but not unique. These male attitudes about female athletes and competition are reminiscent of the ancient Chinese custom of binding young girls' feet. There, females' physical development was restricted to satisfy a cultural norm about femininity; here, female relational development is restricted to satisfy a cultural norm about competition. Both restrictive practices limit all and surely damage some.

If the still predominantly male world of sport and competition becomes more open to the general concepts of relationship and connection, eventually the more specific issues of performance and empowerment will be valued and useful within a culture of what Hill and Oglesby describe as "transformed sport." In such a culture there will be a "shift from endeavor or relationship to one of endeavor and relationship" (Hill & Oglesby, 1995, p. 724).

Abby and Rachel have taught me by their example to value and make more explicit the many and varied relational aspects of my own ongoing love of sports in general and running in particular. To compete within the context of relationships is not only possible–it is desirable. I shall continue to learn from my daughters.

REFERENCES

Belenky, M. F., Clinchy, B. Mc., Goldberger, N. R., & Tarule, J. M. (1986). *Women's ways of knowing: The development of self, voice, and mind.* New York: Basic Books.

Gilligan, C. (1989). Preface: Teaching Shakespeare's sister: Notes from tile underground of female adolescence. In C. Gilligan, T. J. Hanmer, & N. P. Lyons (Eds.), *Making connections: The relational worlds of adolescent girls at Emma Willard School* (pp. 6-29). Cambridge, MA: Harvard University Press.

Hanmer, T. J., Lyons, N. P., & Saltonstall, J. F. (1989). Competencies and visions: Emma Willard girls talk about being leaders. In C. Gilligan, T. J. Hanmer, & N. P. Lyons (Eds.), *Making connections: The relational worlds of adolescent girls at Emma Willard School* (pp. 183-214). Cambridge, MA: Harvard University Press.

Gleason, N., Kaplan, A. G., & Klein R. (1991). Women's self development in late adolescence. In J. V. Jordan, A. G. Kaplan, J. B. Miller, I. P. Stiver, & J. L.

Surrey, *Women's growth in connection: Writings from the Stone Center* (pp. 122-142). New York: The Guilford Press.

Hill, K. L., and Oglesby, C. A. (1995). Gender and sport. In R. N. Singer, M. Murphey, & L. K. Tennant, *Handbook of Research on Sport Psychology* (pp. 718-728). New York: Macmillan Publishing Company.

Stern, L., (1989). Conceptions of separation and connection in female adolescents. In C. Gilligan, T. J. Hanmer, & N. P. Lyons (Eds.), *Makings connections: The relational worlds of adolescent girls at Emma Willard School* (pp. 73-87). Cambridge, MA: Harvard University Press.

Surrey, J. L., (1991a). Relationship and empowerment. In J. V. Jordan, A. G. Kaplan, J. B. Miller, I. P. Stiver, & J. L. Surrey, *Women's growth in connection: Writings from the Stone Center* (pp. 162-180). New York: The Guilford Press.

Surrey, J. L., (1991b). The "self-in-relation": A theory of women's development. In J. V. Jordan, A. G. Kaplan, J. B. Miller, I. P. Stiver, & J. L. Surrey, *Women's growth in connection: Writings from the Stone Center* (pp. 51-66). New York: The Guilford Press.

Softly Strong:
African American Women's Use
of Exercise in Therapy

Ruth L. Hall

SUMMARY. This paper examines how exercise can be integrated into therapy with African American women. Factors that must be considered by the therapist include the client's: (1) attitude toward therapy, exercise, and physical health; (2) socioeconomic status; (3) diagnosis; (4) support system; (5) styles of coping with stress; (6) attitude toward self care; (7) body image; and (8) exposure to realistic role models who exercise. The therapist's sensitivity to an African American cultural context and toward exercise are also critical to successful therapy with African American women. Examples are discussed of using exercise in therapy and professional experiences with African American women. Recommendations are suggested. *[Article copies available for a fee from The Haworth Document Delivery Service: 1-800-342-9678. E-mail address: getinfo@haworth.com]*

The use of exercise in conjunction with traditional forms of psychotherapy, a somewhat novel approach, has been described only occasionally (Hays, 1993, 1994; Sachs & Buffone, 1984; Sime, 1996). Not unlike the literature on traditional therapy, even the literature that exists addresses the use of exercise in psychotherapy with white, middle-class, clients. We cannot assume that the therapeutic approach and intervention with this population works well with all clients (Greene, 1994; Hall, 1995; Hall &

Ruth L. Hall, PhD, is affiliated with the College of New Jersey.

[Haworth co-indexing entry note]: "Softly Strong: African American Women's Use of Exercise in Therapy." Hall, Ruth L. Co-published simultaneously in *The Psychotherapy Patient* (The Haworth Press, Inc.) Vol. 10, No. 3/4, 1998, pp. 81-100; and: *Integrating Exercise, Sports, Movement and Mind: Therapeutic Unity* (ed: Kate F. Hays) The Haworth Press, Inc., 1998, pp. 81-100. Single or multiple copies of this article are available for a fee from The Haworth Document Delivery Service [1-800-342-9678, 9:00 a.m. - 5:00 p.m. (EST). E-mail address: getinfo@haworth.com].

Greene, 1995), as clients bring into therapy a myriad of factors including their culture, their socioeconomic status, and their expectations of therapy. Clearly, several factors influence the efficacy of therapy as well as the introduction of exercise into the therapeutic process.

The purpose of this paper is to examine how exercise can be infused into the therapeutic work with African American women. There is virtually no literature that examines exercise as a therapeutic tool with African American women. Although this article will address basic concerns and potentially successful approaches, we must understand that no one scenario fits all African women, only African American women, or any particular class of women.

Effective integration of exercise into therapy is determined by many factors. Initially, a client's attitude toward therapy, exercise, and physical health (including her susceptibility to heritable diseases such as hypertension and diabetes) must be assessed. Other factors that must be considered include a client's: (1) diagnosis; (2) adherence and motivation to exercise and to continue therapy; (3) support system for exercise and for therapy; (4) exposure to realistic role models who exercise; (5) styles of coping with stress; (6) attitude toward self-care; and (7) body image. Socioeconomic factors, including the amount of discretionary resources (i.e., time and financial resources) available to the client, also influence her commitment to exercise and to therapy. In addition to the therapist's sensitivity to the cultural context relevant to African American women, the therapist's attitude toward exercise is also critical to therapy and exercise adherence: without the therapist's investment in the usefulness of exercise for a client's mental health, the use of exercise will not materialize in the therapeutic process.

The scope of this article does not allow for a full investigation of the roles of culture, internalized racism and sexism, and white privilege in therapy for African American women. I suggest that the reader seek out additional sources for this information (e.g., Boyd-Franklin, 1989; Comas-Diaz & Greene, 1994; Davis, 1981; Dill, 1979; Giddings, 1984; Graham, 1992; Helms, 1991; Hill-Collins, 1991; Lipsky, 1991; McIntosh, 1995; Reid, 1993; Ridley, 1995; Scarr, 1988; Sue, 1991; Tatum, 1987). For those readers who are interested in racial/ethnic issues in athletics, material is also available (Birrell, 1990; Brooks & Althouse, 1993; Duda & Allison, 1990; Hall, 1993, 1996a, 1996b; Jarvie, 1991; Oglesby, 1993).

CULTURE, CLASS, AND GENDER ISSUES IN THERAPY

In order to work effectively with African American women, therapists must appreciate the ways in which culture, gender, and class impact on their clients' lives. Each African American woman has created her own relationship to the African American female experience.

Culture and Femininity

Research on therapy with women of color (Boyd-Franklin, 1991; Childs, 1990; Chin, De La Cancela, & Jenkins, 1993; Espin & Gawelek, 1992) emphasize the need to look at culture for a variety of reasons. Culture provides us with a framework of values and beliefs that serves as a means to organize experience (Betancourt & Lopez, 1993; Hall & Greene, 1995). Unlike race, which is a biologically based definition of difference, culture is a composite of learned behavior that is shared and transmitted by members of a particular society from one generation to the next (Betancourt & Lopez, 1993). Like all women, African American women draw from their rich culture in the development of self-concept and definition. The cultural fabric of African Americans includes: values central to a holistic self-perception (the absence of a definitive split between mind and body experiences); egalitarianism (greater gender equity in heterosexual relationships); spirituality; and the interconnectedness of an extended family, including fictive kin (unrelated individuals who are considered family members).

Personal strength is another dynamic frequently described by African American women. Hall and Bowers (1992) found that African American women, independent of age, marital status, socioeconomic status, and sexual orientation, experience being an African American woman as unique: African American women do not fit or desire to fit the stereotype of femininity. African American women describe themselves as being "softly strong" and recognize that the capacity to be self-sufficient and to be nurtured do not conflict. Moreover, African American women appreciate a more androgenous sexual identity (Comas-Diaz, 1994) and function along a broader spectrum of gender appropriate behavior than their white counterparts.

In addition to her identification with cultural values (i.e., her racial identity) the impact of racism, sexism, and classism can and does compromise a holistic sense of self. Phillips (1996) states that racism is an habitual source of stress for African Americans. Thus, an African American woman, a woman of marginal status, must generate coping skills that create a positive sense of self.

African American Women, Motivation for Therapy, and Diagnosis

African Americans and women of color are understudied populations with regard to the mental health care system, even though they are at greater risk than white women. Not only are mood disorders a primary reason for women to seek therapy (McGrath, Keita, Strickland, & Russo, 1990), the diagnosis of depression is greatest for African Americans below the poverty line (Liu & Yu, 1985). However, many African American women do not access traditional forms of therapy for a variety of reasons. Some African American women feel that personal issues should be discussed only within the extended family rather than disclosed to someone outside the family. Many African American women may believe, accurately or inaccurately, that therapy is not available to them. That "the system" is not to be trusted is another reason not to access therapy. Contact with impersonal governmental agencies and clinics, for low income African Americans, in particular, leaves them skeptical of the "helping professional." Fitting or adhering to traditional therapy parameters may cause problems. For example, low-income African American women may use therapy on an "as needed" basis or may arrive late to sessions. This may lead to miscommunication regarding the intent of keeping appointments: while the therapist feels that she is checking in on the client, the client may perceive that the therapist is checking up on her and terminate therapy prematurely. Finally, the racial and possibly class bias of the therapist is another reason why therapy is not sought out. The client may wonder if the therapist has educated herself, in any way, to the nuances of working with African American female clients.

Given these reasons, a therapist must seek out supplemental interventions that may be more successful and applicable for many women, including African American women. One viable option, especially for the two major diagnoses among women who seek therapy (mood and anxiety disorders, including post-traumatic stress disorder), is exercise (Sime, 1996).

The Therapist-Client Relationship

Once the client has accepted therapy as a means to process her problems, a number of additional factors must be addressed for effective therapy and exercise with African American women. These include: contextual relationships, the therapist as a role model for exercise, and the cultural applicability of exercise.

Contextual in their approach to people and their environment, African American women contextualize therapy as well. Low-income African American women may be particularly invested in contextualizing relationships. Clients may establish a relationship and trust by asking questions about the therapist's personal life (e.g., where she is from) and other information in order to form a contextual grounding with the therapist.

Many times, gaining trust and acceptance from African American clients has little to do with credentials but is more embedded in relatedness, an understanding of family, an appreciation of African American culture, and the importance of connectedness.

Initially, a therapist must conduct a personal inventory and assess her own interest in physical activity. Royak-Schaler and Feldman (1984) found that therapists who believe in and who practice health behaviors are more likely to suggest these behaviors to their clients. If the therapist exercises and shares this information with the client, the client may be more inclined to follow suit. The need for the therapist to model exercise for a client who is an African American woman may be more critical and more functional than for other clients. The African American female therapist would make an ideal role model for African American women. With the exception of Oprah, realistic role models are lacking in the African American women's community, but there may be local role models with whom the client can identify. Seeing other African American women of various sizes and shapes engaged in exercise would make exercise more appealing. If the therapist is not an individual who exercises, other factors in the therapeutic relationship, such as connectedness and relatedness, may be sufficient to encourage a client to exercise.

As therapists, we must use cultural values as they are presented to us and apply them to exercise. For African American women, personal expressiveness (colorful language, demonstrative gestures, candidness) and a sense of community (e.g., group activities) should play a role in therapy and in the introduction of an exercise regimen. For example, group activities such as dance and walking may be more attractive for low-income African American women, in particular, than free weights, swimming or cycling, since these latter activities all involve access to facilities or costly equipment. Dance and aerobic activities can take place in the home or the homes of friends and provide low cost and accessible forms of exercise as well as a social outlet. Given the importance of spirituality in the lives of many African American women, some of these activities could be integrated into their community activities or activities within the church.

Class Issues for African American Women in Therapy

The therapist must distinguish between objective and subjective measures of class. Scholarly definitions notwithstanding, class is an elusive and slippery concept to define. One might question the cultural awareness and ethics of the clinician who uses class and race interchangeably, i.e., seeing African American as synonymous with low income. Although income, occupation, and education are the most frequently used indices of class, for African Americans class is less an issue of income and more an issue of values (e.g., the importance of an education, etc.). Floyd and his associates (1994) determined that a subjective measure of class was more meaningful and relevant for African Americans than an objective measure. Wyche (1996) points out that the therapist must "distinguish between social class, status, and prestige" (p. 40) with African American clients. She states that status outweighs the relevance of class in the African American community, since status denotes respect.

For many communities, including the community where I was raised, blue collar, working-class African American families were perceived as middle-class by the African American community. Also, many African American women who are now middle-class in income were raised in blue collar homes and retain many blue collar values as well. I define class as one's current socioeconomic status, embedded within the context of their family of origin's socioeconomic status.

The therapist must consider class differences that accompany treatment of African American women. Therapists who fail to make these socioeconomic distinctions in their conceptualization of their clients may experience personal dissonance or draw inaccurate conclusions. Low-income African American women have neither the depth nor breadth of resources compared to middle- or upper-class African American women, nor the flexibility and choices such resources provide. Middle-class African Americans are disproportionately represented in high status jobs (e.g., social worker, teacher) which have low salaries (Entwisle & Astone, 1994). Since there is a concentration of African American women in these types of professions, Wyche (1996) states that African American women are not as financially secure as their professions may suggest. Many African American women are financially supporting relatives (a financially needy family member) and there are a significant number of African American women who are raising relatives' children (e.g., nieces, nephews). Additionally, the number of single professional African American women is disproportionally high, particularly among women baby boomers. Relying on a single income can present additional difficulties that may not be present in dual career/dual income households. Class may separate low- and middle-income African American women; however, the realities of oppression specific to the African American experience can override class and create similar barriers that make advancement difficult.

Class, race, and gender influence the choice of physical activity as well. Floyd, Khinew, McGuire, and Noe (1994) found that African Americans' preferred leisure activities, independent of class, were sports (basketball, bowling), health-exercise (aerobics, running), and associations/social activities (dances, parties, organizational affiliations). In contrast, whites preferred fine art (painting, dance), hiking, and outdoor activities (swimming, cycling, sailing). They also found that preferred leisure activities did not differ among white and African American middle-class respondents but did differ with low-income/poor whites and African Americans, particularly between women. While working-class African American women ranked exercise-health 3.5 (out of 14) and sociability 2, white working-class and poor women ranked exercise-health 11 and sociability 14. Middle-class African American and white women ranked exercise-health 6 and 5, respectively. Sociability was ranked much higher for middle-class African Americans (6) than white (12) women. These data complement the cultural value of interconnectedness of African Americans. Sociability is a salient need for African American women and must be taken into consideration in developing an exercise program.

Sallis, Zakarian, Hovell, and Hofsetter (1996) reported that dance was the preferred physical activity for African American adolescents. They also reported that adolescent girls exercise half as much as adolescent boys and that boys selected more strenuous forms of exercise than girls, a finding similar to the Surgeon General's Report on Physical Activity and Health (U.S. Department of Health and Human Services, 1996) which stated that women exercise less than men. They also reported that African American and low-income women exercise less than white women and middle-class women respectively. Additionally, Sallis and his associates found that low-income African American and Latino adolescents had fewer exercise and recreational facilities available to them than white adolescents, independent of class.

Clearly, a therapist must be aware of trends in gender, race, and class preferences of physical activity and the accessibility of facilities. Class may influence the type of exercise that resonates with the client, particularly with regard to financial resources, physical resources, and availability. The therapist must weigh these factors, yet at the same time make no assumptions about a particular client.

EXERCISE AND HOLISTIC HEALTH
IN THE AFRICAN AMERICAN COMMUNITY

Specific concerns that must be addressed with African American women include health-related issues, stress, and body image and size. For each of these issues, exercise and sport participation can provide cost-effective solutions.

Major Health Problems in the African American Community

Leigh (1995) suggested that heritability, poverty, culture, and racism exacerbate health issues for African American women. Hypertension, diabetes, and obesity are major health concerns in the African American community. Genetic predisposition, compounded by culturally influenced dietary habits (i.e., foods high in sodium, sugar, and fat), influences physical well-being for African American women. The National Center for Health Statistics (NCHS) reported that 31% of African American women had hypertension, a rate 1.6 times higher than white women (NCHS, 1995). NCHS also reported that in 1985, 51 per 1,000 African American women vs. 23 per 1,000 white women were diagnosed with hypertension. Diabetes is another major illness in the African American community: African American women are diagnosed twice the rate of diabetes as white women. Obesity, with accompanying high cholesterol levels, is a significant health concern for African American women. Among African American women between the ages of 20 and 74, 50% are overweight (NCHS, 1995) as compared to 34% of white women. Clearly, exercise suggests itself as a strategic intervention in these three major health issues for African American women.

Miller and her colleagues' (1996) study of university students found that African Americans were more concerned about illness rather than about appearance or weight. Thus, health, rather than appearance, may be a more salient motivator for exercise among African American women.

Stress

Although the amount of empirical research available on life stressors for African Americans is limited (Murray & Peacock, 1996), stress remains a significant factor in the lives of African Americans (i.e., Leigh, 1995). African American women are more likely to experience stress-related diseases and die from them (Cope & Hall, 1985) than white women and low-income African American women report the greatest levels of stress (Miller, 1989). Jackson and Sears (1992) and others (Leigh, 1995) agree that class and racism compound and add to the stress felt by African American women. Although code-switching—the capacity to successfully interact fluidly in a bicultural environment—is skillfully honed by African Americans, acculturative stress (Anderson, 1991) persists and compromises the physical and mental health of African Americans. Acculturative stress is encountered when African Americans experience a conflict between their own cultural values and those of the majority community and is part of the daily lives of African Americans. Acculturative stress changes only in intensity. Its pervasiveness is a significant encroachment on the lives of every African American.

Consider living environments, for example. Although the source of stress varies, stress is unavoidable. Neighborhood safety (Sallis et al., 1996; Phillips, 1996) is a factor that impacts of the quality of life for African Americans. Middle-class African Americans who live in an environment where they are only one of few people of color feel a significant amount of stress (Wyche, 1996). In many low-income communities where shootings and other acts of violence are common, G. E. Wyatt (personal communication, February 27, 1992) suggests that the excessive stress warrants a diagnosis of post traumatic stress disorder (PTSD). It must be noted that, independent of class, many women in urban areas cannot engage in the early morning or late evening outdoor exercise for safety reasons. Although exercise can aid in some types of stress reduction, concerns about safety when exercising can exacerbate stress for many urban women.

Body Size and Image

There is both an "upside" and a "downside" in regard to research findings relating to the relationship of African American women and their bodies. Body size and image become noticeable issues in developing an exercise program. Assessing a client's comfort level with her body is a recurring process in therapy. In my experience, body image is frequently a topic in therapy for women, and exercise is most often introduced in the context of weight reduction or maintenance, rather than as a fitness or health related issue. Fitness is most often introduced as a reason for exercise for women who either enjoy exercising or who are not focused on weight reduction. Although magazines that cater to African American women, such as *Essence, Ebony,* and *Heart and Soul,* support and celebrate the spectrum of body types among African American women, the glorification of the physical attributes of white women is presented by society as the accepted norm. That African American women have wide hips, shapely buttocks, a full mouth, and varied hair textures and hues of skin color serves to distinguish African American women—and may also stigmatize them. Many African American women internalize Western standards of beauty that are unrealistic and this may result in a negative body image. According to Greene (1994) racism and internalized oppression take their toll on the body image of African American women. Thus, the greater an African American woman's internalized oppression, the less likely she may be willing to exercise and to "expose" herself.

Despite these circumstances, African American females have a greater level of acceptance and a broader range of body size than do white females (Allan, Mayo, & Michel, 1993; Kumanyika, Wilson, & Guilford-Davenport, 1993; Parker, Nichter, Nichter, Vuckovic, Sims, & Ritenbaugh, 1995). According to Kumanyika and her colleagues, there is less negativity in the African American community regarding obesity and thus, fewer feelings of self-deprecation by African American women, particularly among low income African American women. This, of course, can have negative consequences as well, if a greater acceptance of being overweight results in diminished efforts to practice good nutritional habits.

On a positive note, that African American women have a broader acceptance and greater comfort with their bodies may diminish the presumption that only certain bodies should be seen exercising and donning exercise gear. It is particularly difficult to begin an exercise regimen if one feels excessively self-conscious about her body. In addition, the absence of appropriate and trendy exercise equipment and gear (garments, shoes) may also present a deterrent to exercise. The client may feel that she does not fit in without the right equipment, and may feel conspicuous in how she appears without appropriate attire. Happily, walking and dance require the least equipment, can be purchased on a small budget, and do not necessarily demand form-fitting clothing.

PERSONAL AND PROFESSIONAL EXPERIENCES WITH EXERCISE

Initially, a therapist must conduct a personal inventory and assess her own interest in physical activity. As an African American woman, my experience with exercise and sport has been based primarily on the enjoyment of physical activity. I define myself as a "pre-Title IX recreational athlete." I was President of my high school Girl's Athletic Association. My undergraduate institution had no organized women's sports. However, I have always participated in individual sports or physical activity (swimming, cycling, fitness walking, racquet sports).

Currently, middle-class status enabled me to join a health club with marvelous facilities. I joined primarily to use the pool (I had surgery on my leg and was looking for a low-impact exercise). I have learned to swim and now do laps in the pool, thus experiencing both low impact and a total body workout. Having recently been diagnosed with non-insulin dependent diabetes and mild hypertension (both run in my family), I am hopeful that exercise and dietary changes will result in discontinuing the need for medication. My primary reason to exercise is for enjoyment but I also appreciate that exercise aids in weight reduction, health maintenance, and stress management.

Some clients prefer medication rather than a lifestyle change to modify or to maintain the physiological components of mental and physical health. Medication requires relatively no change in lifestyle and may be perceived as a shortcut to better health. Selling a client on exercise, especially if exercise has not been a factor in her life, is difficult. One may begin with more natural ways of integrating movement that occur through daily activity. Walking versus driving or taking public transportation, or taking the stairs rather than an elevator, are natural ways to begin an exercise program.

My role as a clinician and a sport psychologist with my client athletes is to aid in the optimal execution of their sport. For clients who are not athletes, I do not immediately encourage or recommend an exercise program but I do look for opportunities to interject a discussion on the application of the relationship between physical activity and mental health, particularly for stress management and for affective and anxiety disorders. In my initial intake interview, in addition to the fundamental questions (e.g., chief complaint, medical history, relationship status, education, prior therapy), I include questions about the client's exercise history.

The following vignettes are representative of my experiences in working with African American women in several settings: in private practice, community mental health, and as an officer in an African American psychological organization.

Private Practice Clients

The clients described here specifically sought out an African American female therapist, feeling that cultural similarities were critical to the therapeutic relationship. In addition to their chief complaint, each described the acculturative stress of being an African American in predominantly white professional or academic settings. These clients were either aware of the role of exercise for stress reduction or were introduced to exercise, in part, for stress management.

Paula is a 40-year-old African American female graduate student who I have worked with intermittently for ten years. She began walking for weight reduction and stress management about two years ago. Most recently her chief complaint has been panic attacks stemming in part from her nearly completed doctoral work. She is currently on medication for panic disorder and dysthymia. Throughout, I have encouraged Paula to exercise and told her that exercise would assist with her mood and with stress management. Although health problems have interrupted her exercising, she recently began to exercise again as her physical health improved.

A secondary goal of walking was to have more time to participate in an activity with her mother, as a way to strengthen their relationship. Walking with her mother improved their communication and has also aided Paula in structuring the days she works on her dissertation.

Carron is a 42-year-old African American professional who was seeking support during her transition to a new city and life as an academic after graduate school. She has an established exercise program and uses exercise for enjoyment and as a stress management tool. We discussed how important exercising was to her. She clearly felt better when she exercised, but personal and professional responsibilities frequently compromised her exercise program. The therapist's role regarding exercise in therapy for Carron was to support and monitor, rather than to initiate, a program (Hays, 1993).

Sandra is a 20-year-old college student athlete, a member of a varsity team at her university. For Sandra, exercise was well integrated into her lifestyle. Exercise maintained her level of fitness and provided an outlet for school related stress. Unlike most of my clients, Sandra's chronic injuries jeopardized her athletic career and she was forced to cut back on her exercise program. Eventually Sandra resigned from her team and participated in athletics at an intramural and recreational level. Our goal was to make the transition as smooth as possible and to help her mourn the loss she experienced letting go of her dreams and aspirations of becoming an Olympic athlete. For Sandra, her faith served as a resource and comforted her transition, indicative of the central role of spirituality in the lives of many African Americans.

Brenda is a 45-year-old professional African American woman who entered therapy to discuss her current relationship and some unresolved issues concerning her family of origin. Although Brenda was a large woman, she was not experiencing any health-related problems. She wanted to lose weight and had never exercised on a regular basis. Brenda joined a health club in her neighborhood but was never able to consistently exercise. Efforts to provide support for her desire to "work out" and to reduce job induced stress were not helpful. For Brenda, exercise was not a priority, even though talking about her desire to exercise remained relatively constant.

To summarize, my experiences with using exercise in therapy are mixed. Even so, I continue to ask each new client about her use of and reasons for exercise.

Experiences in a Community Mental Health Center

In my position as Associate Director of a Philadelphia community mental health center, I worked primarily with a predominantly low income African American population, many of whom could not afford membership fees at a health facility or local YMCA. My caseload was primarily women and children. The women from the community entered therapy for a variety of reasons, including family, child and marital problems, and personal problems exacerbated by classism, racism, sexism, and their economic status. Most of the women had no regular exercise program. Many of the women did not receive support for seeking therapy or for beginning and maintaining an exercise regimen. They were frequently the only ones in their family who used therapy and the only ones who exercised.

As the Associate Director, I was able to persuade the administration to purchase a few pieces of exercise equipment for the center: a universal weight machine, an exercise pad, and a stationary bicycle. The equipment was in one room in the building and the women could come and go as they pleased. I found that exercising with my clients was an optimal means of initiating an exercise program. Since discretionary time and finances were problems, combining therapy and exercise made good use of both resources. While some of the women came to the clinic to exercise in addition to therapy, the need for support and for modeling was evident.

I found that organizing the women into a small support group was helpful. The women were able to encourage one another's exercise goals, and the group experience expanded their network of women who were interested in exercise. Culturally, the sense of community common in the African American experience was beneficial to sustaining the group experience. The group was most active when I was directly involved. When I was unable to meet consistently with group members individually or collectively, the group disbanded. Overall, I would describe the experience as modestly successful.

The children who came in for therapy at the community health center were more likely than adults to embrace exercise and physical activity. Physical activity and play therapy are complementary processes in therapy with children. Because of the condition of the neighborhood playground (glass covered surfaces), initially I played with the children within the facility. When the playground was cleaned we would take kickballs, basketballs, jump ropes, and other gross motor devices to the playground. Both the attention and the activity generated an enhanced therapist-client relationship and provided a forum to discuss their concerns. Play was an ideal means to work psychotherapeutically with children, and I reinforced the function of exercise through play.

Experiences in a Professional Organization

Similarly, I employed the concept of community as a means to foster interest in exercise. When I was the president of the Delaware Valley Association of Black Psychologists in 1982, I initiated a monthly exercise activity built into the organization's calendar year. My goal was to encourage professionals' interest in holistic health and to provide a shared social experience for the association. The activities included cycling, ice skating, horseback riding, and bowling. The monthly activities were announced at each general meeting and all members were invited to attend. I selected a variety of activities, hoping to create interest with as many members as possible. The activities met with modest response by the membership and those who participated enjoyed the opportunity to connect with other individuals within the organization. I feel that it is essential to generate a therapist's interest in physical activity in order to get clients invested in physical activity.

Professional Colleagues' Experiences

I have two professional African American colleagues who have begun to integrate exercise into their lives, their therapy, and their teaching. They both began to exercise consistently after age 40. Both are seasoned clinicians with more than 10 years of clinical experience. Both had strong racial identities, accepted their racial body types (hips, buttocks) and did not perceive exercise as a means to meet the social "norm" of a white female body type. Both women used exercise as a tool for stress management but they differed in additional incentives to exercise. While Dr. D. was concerned with weight maintenance, Dr. M. was motivated by health-related concerns.

Dr. D. stated that exercise can be used as a "forum to tackle life issues." She feels that exercise and depression are related in that both "push the limits." For better and for worse, each uses the cognitive technique of self talk to maintain itself. Initially, Dr. D. did not bring up exercising regularly to her clients and waited for them to approach exercise as a topic. However, as she became more aware of the benefits of exercise for her own stress management, mood, and weight maintenance, she began to introduce the suggestion of exercise into therapy, particularly for clients diagnosed with dysthymic disorder. She felt that depressed clients, especially, could make the transition from using their cognitive skills in maintaining their depression to using those skills to develop an exercise program. Self-talk works!

A second colleague, Dr. M., began to exercise regularly for health reasons. When I first met her in 1985, she did not exercise and stated, "I don't want to do anything that makes me sweat." She had taken up walking in spurts over the years but had not walked for exercise with any consistency. She eventually began walking for weight reduction and her exercise was reinforced by her former therapist who was an avid runner. Dr. M. stated that she had initially ignored her therapist's attempts to encourage her to exercise because her therapist was a runner, something in which Dr. M. had no interest. She began to walk more consistently in 1994 for several reasons. First and foremost was her health: Dr. M. was diagnosed with hypertension and diabetes. Dr. M. now fitness walks approximately 20 miles each week and is walking at a faster pace. She has become interested in cross training and purchased a Nordic Track and, most recently, a stationary bicycle. Dr. M. has set a goal of maintaining an exercise regimen for a year. "I have a cognitive mo-jo working now. I will reevaluate my status in a year and decide then whether or not I should continue." Dr. M. stated that she was more likely to introduce exercise to her clients and to her students as a stress management tool. She is more cognizant of benefits of exercise and has a greater appreciation of an exercise regimen.

CONCLUDING REMARKS

There are many ways in which a therapist can be successful in using exercise with therapy for African American women. The list that follows recaps some of the mechanisms that can make exercise in therapy a reality:

- Value the role of exercise in self-care and holistic health
- As part of your identifying data, ask client about her exercise regimen
- Have magazines and pictures in your waiting area that show women (including women of color) exercising and participating in physical activities
- Work within the culture, class, and gender schemas
- Appreciate the limitations of freedom of movement for women in urban settings
- Explain that there are a variety of exercise activities for clients and that running is not the only exercise program

- Encourage the client to integrate exercise as part of her lifestyle for health and for fitness
- Inform the client that exercise helps the management of stress, sexual tension, insomnia, and health problems, and also promotes a sense of well being, enhances self esteem, and fosters self confidence
- Encourage the client to maintain a log/journal of her physical activity
- Help the client set realistic goals
- Use bibliotherapy and suggest books and articles that focus on the benefits of exercise
- Discuss performance enhancement techniques. They can be used within therapy for depression (e.g., cognitive behavioral approaches) and stress management
- Discuss exercise adherence and lapses as natural phenomena
- Discuss the social benefits of exercise (group activities with friends or family members)

A Prescription for Therapists

Therapists must be aware that African Americans underuse therapy, relying instead on community-based outlets for mental health concerns, such as the church and the extended community. Thus, African American women may have to be sold on the efficacy of both therapy and exercise as useful intervention tools for depression, health concerns and stress.

It is imperative that therapists examine their own biases about healthy behavior and not make unwarranted assumptions about their clients based on the client's gender, age, race, class, or body type or size. Unconscious racism, classism, and sexism can work against the therapist. Rather than presume or promote specific forms of exercise, therapists need to work out probable types with their clients. For example, therapists should not assume that all African American females, independent of class, like rap music or dislike classical music to accompany their exercise.

Thus, when working with African American women, therapists must assess the overt and covert contributors to stress and its cumulative effects, particularly for the "softly strong" African American woman. Stress management, rather than weight reduction or fitness, may well be the optimal means to encourage African American women to exercise.

Race, ethnicity and gender are interactive variables for African American women: both influence their perception of and interaction with their world and a sense of themselves. Artificially separating these aspects of the self diminishes and invalidates one's experience as an African American woman. For true validation, we must acknowledge the roles of race, ethnicity and gender schemas in their lives. Whether as individuals or as a group, women who integrate exercise into their physical well-being are actively participating in self-care and in holistic health. Bringing the discussion of exercise into therapy and the support of its inclusion in clients' lives are ways of establishing a connection with clients that is holistic, non-threatening and contextual.

REFERENCES

Allan, J. D., Mayo, K., & Michel, Y. (1993). Body size values of white and Black women. *Research in Nursing & Health, 16,* 323-333.

Anderson, L. P. (1991). Acculturative stress: A theory of relevance to Black Americans. *Clinical Psychology Review, 11,* 685-702.

Betancourt, H. & Lopez, S. R. (1993). The study of culture, ethnicity and race in American psychology. *American Psychologist, 48,* 629-637.

Birrell, S. (1989). Racial relations theories and sport: Suggestions for a more critical analysis. *Sociology of Sport Journal, 8,* 212-227.

Boyd-Franklin, N. (1991). Recurrent themes in the treatment of African American women in group therapy. *Women in Therapy, 11* (2). 25-40.

Boyd-Franklin, N. (1989). *Black families in therapy: A multisystems approach.* New York: Guilford Press.

Brooks, D. & Althouse, R. (1993). *Racism in college athletics: The African-American athlete.* Morgantown, WV: Fitness Information Technology, Inc.

Childs, E. K. (1990). Therapy, feminist ethics, and the community of color with particular emphasis on the treatment of black women. In H. Lerman & N. Porter (Eds.). *Feminist ethics in psychotherapy* (pp. 195-203). New York: Springer.

Chin, J. L., De La Cancela, V. & Jenkins, Y. (1993). Themes in psychotherapy with diverse populations. In L. J. Chin, V. De La Cancela, & Y. Jenkins (Eds.). *Diversity in psychotherapy* (pp. 171-182). Westport, CT: Praeger.

Comas-Diaz, L. (1994). An integrative approach. In L. Comas-Diaz & B. Greene (Eds.). *Women of color: Integrating ethnic and gender identities in psychotherapy* (pp. 287-318). New York, NY: Guilford Press.

Comas-Diaz, L. & Greene, B. (Eds.). *Women of color: Integrating ethnic and gender identities in psychotherapy.* New York, NY: Guilford Press.

Cope, N. R. & Hall, H. R. (1985). The health status of Black women in the United States: Implications for health psychology and behavioral medicine. *Sage, 2,* 20-24.

Davis, A. (1981). *Women race and class.* New York: Random House.

Dill, B. T. (1979). The dialectics of black womanhood. *Signs, 4,* 545-555.

Duda, J. L. & Allison, M. T. (1990). Cross-cultural analysis in exercise and sport psychology: A void in the field. *Journal of Sport and Exercise Psychology, 12,* 114-131.

Entwisle, D. & Astone, N. (1994). Some practical guidelines for measuring youth's race/ethnicity and socioeconomic status. *Child Development, 65,* 1521-1540.

Espin, O. & Gawelek, M. A. (1992). Women's diversity: Ethnicity, race, class, and gender in theories of feminist psychology. In L. Brown and M. Ballou (Eds.). *Personality and psychopathology: Feminist appraisals* (pp. 88-107). New York: Guilford Press.

Floyd, M. F., Shinew, K. J., McGuire, F. A., & Noe, F. P. (1994). Race, class, and leisure activity preferences: Marginality and ethnicity revisited. *Journal of Leisure Research 26,* 158-173.

Giddings, P. (1984). *When and where I enter: The impact of race and sex in America.* New York: Bantam Books.

Graham, S. (1992). "Most of the subjects were white and middle class": Trends in published research of African Americans in selected APA journals, 1970-1989. *American Psychologist, 47,* 629-639.

Greene, B. (1994). Diversity and difference: The issues of race in feminist therapy. In M. P. Mierkin (ed.). *Women in context: Toward a feminist reconstruction of psychotherapy* (pp. 333-35 1). New York: Guilford Publications.

Hall, R. L. (1996a). Ethnic identify and cross racial experiences of college athletes. Unpublished masters thesis. Temple University, Philadelphia.

Hall, R. L. (1996b). Sweating it out: Women and sport. In J. C. Chrisler, C. Golden, & P. Rosee (Eds.). *Lectures in the psychology of women* (pp. 89-102). New York: McGraw-Hill.

Hall, R. L. (1995). Barriers, Assumptions, and Expectations: Issues of Class and Race for African American Women. Presentation at the Association for Women in Psychology. Indianapolis, Indiana.

Hall, R. L. (1993). Racial Identity and Team Racial Composition of Women's Varsity Basketball Players. Presentation at the American Psychological Association. Toronto, Canada.

Hall, R. L. & Greene, B. (1995). Cultural competency and feminist family therapy: An ethical mandate. *Journal of Feminist Family Therapy, 6,* 2-11.

Hall, R. L. & Bowers, C. D. (1992). Afrocentricity and womanhood. American Psychological Association Centennial Conference. Washington, DC.

Hays, K. F. (1994). Running therapy: Special characteristics and therapeutic issues of concern. *Psychotherapy 31,* 725-734.

Hays, K. F. (1993). The use of exercise in psychotherapy. In L. VandeCreek, S. Knapp, & T. L. Jackson (Eds.). *Innovations in clinical practice: A source book* (Vol. 12) (pp. 155-168). Sarasota, FL: Professional Resource Press.

Hays, K. F. & Smith, R. J. (1996). Incorporating sport and exercise psychology into clinical practice. In J. L. Van Raalte & B. W. Brewer (Eds.). *Exploring sport and exercise in psychology* (413-430). Washington, DC: American Psychological Association.

Helms, J. (Ed.). (1991). *Black and white racial identity: Theory. research and practice.* New York: Greenwood Press.

Hill-Collins, P. (1991). *Black feminist thought: Knowledge, consciousness, and the politics of empowerment.* New York: Routlege.

Horton, J. A. (Ed.). (1992). *The women's health data book: A profile of women's health in the United States*. Washington, DC: Jacobs Institute of Women's Health.

Jackson, J. J. (1973). Black women in a racist society. In C.V. Willie, B.M. Kramer and B. S. Brown (Eds.). *Racism and mental health* (pp. 185-268). Pittsburgh: University of Pittsburgh Press.

Jackson, A. P. & Sears, S. J. (1992). Applications of an africentric worldview in reducing stress for African American women. *Journal of Counseling and Development, 71*, 184-190.

Jarvie, G. (Ed.). (1991). *Sport, racism, and ethnicity*. Philadelphia: Falmer Press.

Kumanyika, S., Wilson, J. F., & Guilford-Davenport, M. (1993). Weight-related attitudes and behaviors of black women. *Journal of the American Dietetic Association, 93*, 416-422.

Leigh, W. A. (1995). The health of African American women. In D. L. Adams, (ed.). Health issues for women of color: A cultural diversity perspective. (pp. 112-132). Thousand Oaks, CA: Sage.

Lipsky, S. (1991). Internalized Oppression. In G. L. Mallon (Ed.). *Resisting racism: An action guide* (pp. 94-99). San Francisco: National Association of Black and White Men Together.

Liu W. T. & Yu, E. S. (1985). Ethnicity, mental health, and the urban delivery system. In L. Maldonado, & J. Moore (Eds.). *Urban ethnicity in the United States* (211-247). Beverly Hills, CA: Sage.

Mays, V. M., Caldwell, C. H. & Jackson, J. S. (1995). Mental health symptoms and service utilization patterns of help-seeking among African American women. In H. W. Neighbors and J. S. Jackson (Eds). *Mental health in Black America* (pp. 161-176). Thousand Oaks, CA: Sage.

McGrath, E., Keita, G. P., Strickland, R. R., & Russo, N.F. (1990). *Women and depression: Risk factors and treatment issues*. Washington, DC: American Psychological Association.

McIntosh, P. (1995). White privilege and male privilege. In M.L. Anderson & P. Hill Collins (Eds.). *Race, class & gender* (pp. 76-99). Belmont, CA: Wadsworth.

Miller, K. J., Gleaves, D. H., Hirsch, T. G., Corbett, C. C., Snow, A. C., & Green, B. A. (1996, August). University Students' Body Images: Comparisons by Race/Ethnicity and Gender. Poster session presented at the American Psychological Association, Toronto, Canada.

Miller, S. M. (1989). Race in the health of America. In D. P. Wallis (Ed.). *Health policies and Black Americans* (pp. 500-531). New Brunswick, NJ: Transaction.

Murray, C. B. & Peacock (1996). A model-free approach to the study of subjective well-being. In H. W. Neighbors and J. S. Jackson (Eds). *Mental health in Black America* (pp. 14-26). Thousand Oaks, CA: Sage.

National Center for Health Statistics (NCHS)(1995). *Health, United States, 1994*. Hyattsville, MD: Public Heath Service.

Oglesby, C. (1993). Issues of sport and racism: Where is the white in the rainbow coalition? In D. D. Brooks, R. C. Althouse (Eds.). *Racism in college athletics* (pp. 252-267). Morgantown, VA: F.I.T. Inc.

Parker, S., Nichter, M., Nichter, M., Vuckovic, N., Sims, C., Ritenbaugh, C.

(1995). Body image and weight concerns among African American and white adolescent females: Differences that make a difference. *Human Organization 54*, 103-114.

Phillips, G. Y. (1996). Stress and residential well-being. In H. W. Neighbors and J. S. Jackson (Eds). *Mental health in Black America* (pp. 27-44). Thousand Oaks, CA: Sage.

Reid, P. T. (1993). Poor women in psychological research: Shut up and shut out. *Psychology of Women Quarterly. 17*, 133-150.

Ridley, C. R. (1995). *Overcoming unintentional racism in counseling and therapy: A practitioner's guide to intentional intervention*. Thousand Oaks, CA: Sage.

Royak-Schaler, R. & Feldman, R. H. L. (1984). Health behaviors of psychotherapists. *Journal of Clinical Psychology. 40*, 705-710.

Russell, G. M. (1996). Internalized classism: the role of class in the development of self. *Women & Therapy. 18(3/4)*, 59-72.

Sachs, M. L. & Buffoon, G. W. (Eds.). (1984). *Running as therapy: An integrated approach*. Lincoln: University of Nebraska Press.

Sallis, J. F., Zakarian, J. M., Hovell, M. F., & Hofsetter, C. R. (1996). Ethnic, socioeconomic, and sex differences in physical activity among adolescents. *Journal of Clinical Epidemiology, 49*, 125-134.

Scarr, S. (1988). Race and gender as psychological variables. *American Psychologist, 43*, 56-59.

Secundy, M. G. (1995). Ethical Issues in Research. In D. L. Adams (Ed.). *Health issues for women of color: A cultural diversity perspective* (pp. 228-238). Thousand Oaks, CA: Sage.

Sime, W. (1996). Guidelines for clinical applications of exercise therapy for mental health. In J. L. Van Raalte & B. W. Brewer (Eds.). *Exploring sport and exercise in psychology* (159-187). Washington, DC: American Psychological Association.

Sue, D. W. (1991). *Counseling the culturally different: Theory & practice* (2nd ed.). New York: John Wiley and Sons.

Tatum, B. (1987). *Assimilation blues: Black families in a white community*. Northampton, MA: Greenwood.

U.S. Department of Health and Human Services (1996). *Physical activity and health: A report of the Surgeon General*. Atlanta, GA: U. S. Department of Health and Human Services, Centers for Disease Control and Prevention, National Center for Chronic Disease Prevention and Health Promotion.

Women's Sports Foundation (1989, October 27). Minorities in sports. The effect of varsity sports participation on the social, educational, and career mobility of minority students. *The Women's Sports Foundation Report*. New York: Women's Sports Foundation.

Women's Sports Foundation (1994, March 1). *Women's sports facts*. New York: Women's Sports Foundation.

Wyche, K. F. (1996). Conceptualizations of social class in African American women: Congruence of client and therapist definitions. *Women & Therapy, 18(3/4)*, 35-44.

SPORT PSYCHOLOGY CONSULTATION

Working in Competitive Sport: What Coaches and Athletes Want Psychologists to Know

Judy L. Van Raalte

SUMMARY. Work with competitive athletes is rewarding and challenging. Understanding the unique aspects of the elite sport environment can enhance psychological consultation. This paper begins with several case examples, then background characteristics common to many athletes are described, e.g., early involvement in sport participation, reliance on sport specific behavioral norms. It is suggested that paying particular attention to athletes' sport history, time demands, and sport characteristics will increase satisfaction with sport psychology services. The important role that coaches and the media play in athletes' lives is also described. Discussion of these points is essential because psychologists who gain familiarity with elite sport environments will better serve their competitive athlete

Judy L. Van Raalte, PhD, is affiliated with the Center for Performance Enhancement and Applied Research, Department of Psychology, Springfield College, Springfield, MA 01109.

[Haworth co-indexing entry note]: "Working in Competitive Sport: What Coaches and Athletes Want Psychologists to Know." Van Raalte, Judy L. Co-published simultaneously in *The Psychotherapy Patient* (The Haworth Press, Inc.) Vol. 10, No. 3/4, 1998, pp. 101-110; and: *Integrating Exercise, Sports, Movement and Mind: Therapeutic Unity* (ed: Kate F. Hays) The Haworth Press, Inc., 1998, pp. 101-110. Single or multiple copies of this article are available for a fee from The Haworth Document Delivery Service [1-800-342-9678, 9:00 a.m. - 5:00 p.m. (EST). E-mail address: getinfo@haworth.com].

101

clients in need of psychological services. *[Article copies available for a fee from The Haworth Document Delivery Service: 1-800-342-9678. E-mail address: getinfo@haworth.com]*

THE COMPETITIVE ATHLETE

In many ways, working with competitive athletes is the glamorous side of applied sport psychology. For both athletes and sport psychologists, championships, victories, and media attention all contribute to the glory. However, applied work with competitive athletes can also be challenging for sport psychologists. Odd hours, performance demands, notoriety, limitations in access to athletes, and media relations can all make productive work more difficult.

The purpose of this paper is to describe aspects of competitive sport that are particularly relevant for providing psychological services to competitive athletes. The paper begins with several case examples highlighting some of the situations that a psychologist might encounter working with competitive athletes. The next section focuses on specific aspects of the sport environment that are important for sport psychology service delivery.

CASE EXAMPLES

Case #1

John is a professional football player who has recently been working with a sport psychologist on pain management techniques. John has been an avid learner and has found a number of techniques that are useful to him. As the sessions progress, the sport psychologist learns that John is being encouraged by his coaches to use these techniques to avoid medical intervention for a serious injury. The sport psychologist provides support for John, who, although able to "play through" the pain, wants to seek treatment for his injury.

Case #2

Dave is a member of his college track team and hopes to eventually qualify for the Olympics. Lately, he has seemed somewhat anxious and depressed. Dave's coach has recommended that Dave meet with a local sport psychologist who has been hired to work with the team. In their first meeting, Dave tells the sport psychologist that he is frustrated with the way the coach runs the team. Dave adds that he would like to learn to speak up for himself. The sport psychologist works with Dave, using role play and a variety of other techniques. Dave reports that he feels better about his ability to address his coach. Shortly thereafter, the coach contacts the sport psychologist and angrily complains about Dave's "mouthing off." The coach threatens to throw Dave off the team if he does not shape up his attitude.

Case #3

Janice began her involvement in competitive archery at a relatively young age and had great success in the sport. Over the years, Janice has established herself as one of the top competitors in the United States. Janice's goals include performing well "locally" as well as at the international level. Janice began meeting with a sport psychologist because she wanted to "go the extra mile" necessary to reach the highest level of her sport. The sessions have been useful to Janice in enhancing her concentration and confidence and she has asked the sport psychologist to travel with her to competitions so that their work will not be interrupted. The offer to continue work with Janice is enticing, but travelling with Janice would require the sport psychologist to reschedule other clients and manage various time and money issues.

Case #4

To help identify those athletes who will perform best as professional athletes, the team management has contracted with a psychologist to do psychological testing. All the athletes sign consent forms agreeing to share the results of their tests with the team's management. After testing is completed, Alysha changes her mind and asks that her test results be kept confidential. The management of the team, which is paying for the tests, demands to see the results of all tests performed.

These case examples provide an overview of some of the situations that can occur when sport psychologists work with competitive athletes. In the case of John, techniques introduced by the sport psychologist to help manage pain are being used in ways that may cause John physical harm. Unlike many work places, the arena of competitive sport may actually encourage or foster risky behavior. For Dave, psychological intervention has enhanced his personal growth but has led him into conflict with his elite sport opportunities. The power of the coach in competitive sport should not be underestimated. In the case of Janice, a successful outcome has led to her desire to travel with her sport psychologist. Janice's situation highlights the scheduling, time, and money difficulties that can arise for sport psychologists working with competitive athletes. Finally, in the case of Alysha, conflict between the person receiving services and those paying for services has created an ethical dilemma with confidentiality issues. Familiarity with the sport environment can be useful in preventing such problems from arising.

These case examples illustrate some of the complexities for sport psychologists working in the competitive sport environment. Discussion of background factors that can be useful to understand when working with competitive athletes are presented in more detail below.

WORKING IN COMPETITIVE SPORT (WHAT COACHES AND ATHLETES WANT PSYCHOLOGISTS TO KNOW)

Although work with competitive athletes is similar to work with other clients, it differs in significant ways which are highlighted here and described in more detail below. For example, most competitive athletes have been highly involved in their sport from childhood. Thus, they typically identify strongly with the athlete role (Brewer, Van Raalte, & Linder, 1993). Many competitive athletes have developed an intense desire to succeed in sport, an "anything to win" attitude. The closed nature of the competitive sport environment can reduce the likelihood that athletes will have contact with outside experiences and avenues of social support. Pressure on competitive athletes can be intensified by media attention. This scrutiny, however, may increase competitive athletes' concerns about the mental health stigma that applies to those who seek psychological services.

The Importance of Sport to Athletes

For many, the dream of being an outstanding athlete begins in childhood and permeates all areas of life (e.g., academic, health, social). Parents who are strongly invested in sport may hire academic tutors so that their children can spend less time in school and get extra practice in sport, may send their children to specialized sport academies, and even "overlook" anabolic steroid use (Hellstedt, 1995; Weinberg & Gould, 1995). Parents' and coaches' desire to help young athletes achieve competitive success can contribute to a strong task focus but can also be a burden on developing children.

Petitpas and his colleagues have suggested that competitive athletes may lag in psychosocial development relative to their nonathlete peers (Pearson & Petitpas, 1990; Petitpas, 1978; Petitpas & Champagne, 1988). As athletes mature, their intense involvement in competitive sport may become their primary focus and they therefore may not engage in the quest for self that characterizes full identity development. The strong commitment to sport can promote a "do it at any cost" mentality. Indeed, intercollegiate athletes who identify strongly and exclusively with the athlete role are more likely than other athletes to say that they would give up 10 years of their lives to earn an Olympic gold medal (Hale, 1995).

Thus, for many competitive athletes, sport is something more than "just a game," it is their identity. Competitive athletes, both male and female, are more likely than nonathletes to strongly endorse such statements as "Most of my friends are athletes," "I would be very depressed if I were injured and could not compete in sport," and "Sport is the only important thing in my life" (Brewer et al., 1993). By providing the focus and motivation necessary to perform at a high level, a strong, albeit narrow, athletic identity can be beneficial for an athlete's involvement in competitive sport (Brewer et al., 1993).

A strong athletic identity may enhance an athlete's interest in improving performance through a number of avenues including consulting a sport psychologist. Consulting with a sport psychologist may be especially useful for athletes who are injured or who go into a performance slump. Because sport is such a central part of their lives, these athletes may lack coping resources such as interests and/or sources of social support outside sport. Coaches may have little time to devote to injured athletes or those performing marginally, needing to focus instead on those who are actively competing. Some athletes may feel a sense of abandonment in this situation and may also be more likely than other athletes to become depressed (Brewer, 1993).

Clearly, it behooves sport psychologists to recognize the centrality of sport in competitive athletes' lives. For many competitive athletes, sport is a job, an identity, and a social role.

The "Just Do It" Norms of Competitive Sport

Competitive sport environments have different norms and standards of behavior from those of society at large. These norms have developed in high pressure closed environments. Competitive sport is pervaded with a "just do it" mentality. Although high level competitive athletes may take into account the value of incorporating some rest periods in their training, they generally value a "more is better" approach. Health and competence are at a premium. Any sign of weakness can be seen as a failing, a lack of ability and/or a lack of commitment (Petrie, 1993).

Some athletes may be hesitant to work with a sport psychologist because of the response they anticipate receiving. Male sports fans and college students have been found to derogate athletes who consult sport psychologists (Linder, Brewer, Van Raalte, & DeLange, 1991). On the brighter side, athletes who consult sport psychologists are not derogated by their fellow athletes (Van Raalte, Brewer, Brewer, & Linder, 1992). This suggests that there is some acceptance of the need for sport psychology services among competitive athletes. Awareness of the norms of competitiveness in the sport world can facilitate the building of effective relationships among sport psychologists, athletes, and coaches.

The Closed Nature of Competitive Sport

Working with athletes in the competitive sport environment can be more difficult than working with people in other environments because of the controls exerted on athletes' lives by their coaches. Coaches are instrumental in determining the sport opportunities of their athletes and often encourage their athletes to excellence by demanding that the athletes "give 110%" to the team. Coaches may have policies restricting the foods that athletes can eat, the activities that they can be involved in prior to competition (e.g., no sex before the big game), and the people with whom they associate. Control can be particularly important to coaches because their jobs may depend on the ability to attain winning records.

Sport psychologists need to be sensitive to the external career pressures that affect coaches. Working with coaches to establish a balance of power with athletes may be possible in some situations. In other cases, the sport psychologists may have to "let it go" and work within the existing athletic system.

There is no easy way into the closed world of competitive sport. Sport psychologists who know someone on the "inside" clearly have an advantage. Reading books and watching practices and competitions can facilitate the transition from outsider to insider. Patience and persistence are both useful tools in entering the sport arena.

Meeting with Competitive Athletes

The strength of the mental health stigma makes it likely that competitive athletes will have some concerns when they first meet with a sport psychologist. Although each athlete and practitioner is different, there are a number of things that can be done to put athletes more at ease. Four techniques (gathering a sport history, being aware of time constraints, carefully selecting assessment instruments, and limiting use of technical psychological language) are described in more detail below.

"Understand my sport history, understand me." Involvement in sport forms the core of many competitive athletes' identity. Gathering a sport history, in addition to the usual historical information, is one way that a sport psychologist can signal to an athlete that sport involvement is considered important (Taylor & Schneider, 1992). For example, a sport psychologist could inquire about how an athlete began in sport, how long they have been competing, what their strengths and weaknesses are, what they like best about their sport, and what their current sport concerns are.

Time constraints. Although gathering extensive information is important, it should be noted that competitive athletes often have limited time for consultation. Some competitive athletes may be so busy with practice, weight training, and jobs and/or school that they do not have time for consultation during the competitive season (Andersen, 1996). Other athletes' schedules are such that they can meet with a sport psychologist only if the sport psychologist travels to the site of practices or competitions. Situations such as those with Janice (case #3) can pose particular scheduling and financial difficulties. Sport psychologists should be familiar enough with the sport environment to anticipate these challenges. For example, if the sport psychologist decides to travel with Janice, then meetings "on the road" should be planned. Privacy issues, housing arrangements, and an appropriate place for sessions should all be clarified. Coordinating details of consultation and travel with the coach may also be important. Some sport psychologists resolve these difficulties by making their own travel arrangements and paying their own way to a limited number of competitions. Other sport psychologists restrict their travel to limit potential countertransferential issues and dependency problems.

Assessment. In situations where time concerns loom large, use of general assessment instruments may not be appropriate (Gardner, 1995). Some athletes may feel that the sport psychologist does not understand them if they are required to complete long, seemingly meaningless questionnaires. Unless sport psychologists carefully explain the purpose of the tests, athletes may choose to terminate consultation before it even really starts. In other situations, such as that with Alysha described in case #4, athletes may feel that the results of general tests should not be shared with others. Coaches, on the other hand, may feel that it is their right to have access to important information that they are paying for and that can help enhance the success of their careers. In situations where the coaching staff and/or management is paying to have the competitive athletes tested, sport psychologists can have a difficult time identifying who exactly their client is and how confidentiality should be maintained. Clear discussion of these issues and development of an appropriate plan with all parties involved can reduce the likelihood that such problems will arise.

Learn the language. Finally, athletes are more likely to continue in consultation with sport psychologists who understand and use the terminology and rules of the sport in which their clients participate. For example, an athlete may participate in a football *game,* a swim *meet,* or a tennis *match.* Asking a football player if he has a meet this week can lead to a loss of credibility. As athletes thrive in a physical culture, they may more easily understand and identify with nontechnical language related to health rather than pathology. Although athletes should feel free to ask questions if they do not understand the technical terminology being used, they may be hesitant to speak up and appear to be "dumb jocks." Clearly, this is not the case for all athletes, but it is important to be sensitive to the limited familiarity that some athletes have with psychological language.

Treatment

Treatment of competitive athletes depends on the theoretical orientation of the practitioner as well as the needs of the client. Nonetheless, certain general treatment factors apply to work with this population. Sport psychologists should be aware of the efficacy of behavioral approaches with many athletes, the difficulties of scheduling long-term treatment, the costs and benefits of involving coaches in the treatment process, and the challenges inherent in dealing with interested media personnel.

Competitive athletes often lead very structured lives. Part of their success has probably depended on their ability to balance personal, sport, work, and school demands. Although many competitive athletes are no longer enrolled in school programs, most have been involved in school work during some portion of their competitive career. The need to simultaneously organize a number of time-consuming demands has helped many competitive athletes become familiar with goal setting techniques. Sport training focuses on specific behaviors leading to specific outcomes (e.g., "if you do more sprints in practice, you will run faster in competition"). Many competitive athletes are good candidates for cognitive behavioral interventions because of their understanding of the interrelationships among cognitive factors (e.g., concentration, confidence), affect, and performance. Clearly, athletes differ in their preferences, interests, and capabilities, so the specific treatment should be matched to the athlete's problem, needs, and practitioner's expertise.

Some sport psychologists have found that a strong allegiance with the team coach is a prerequisite to working with a team, while others have found a close tie to the coach to be problematic (Baillie & Ogilvie, 1996). Because coaches are often central to athletes' lives, involvement of coaches can facilitate treatment. Some sport psychologists work with athletes on the playing field, court, etc. It is not atypical for an athlete to request that a sport psychologist attend a practice or competition. For these situations, coach involvement and cooperation is essential. If a coach is dissatisfied with the athlete's progress, as in the case of Dave (case #2), the coach may contribute to the demise of the consulting relationship. Recognizing that athletes function within a sport system in which the coach has primary control can be useful for sport psychologists beginning to work with competitive sport teams. Coaches generally care about their individual athletes. At the same time, they are also responsible for a number of athletes, are often extremely busy with the coaching and administrative demands of their jobs, and are necessarily focused on winning. Obviously, sport psychologists should work with coaches, treat them with respect, and be sure not to overstep boundaries and create additional problems for coaches.

If the coach does become involved with athlete treatment, boundaries can be further complicated by the media. Coaches do not have the same ethical confidentiality guidelines that psychologists do. Educating coaches about confidentiality issues can be important. Confidential psychological information that is leaked to the media can result in the termination of the athlete-sport psychologist relationship.

CONCLUSION

Providing psychological services to competitive athletes can be a challenging and rewarding experience. Awareness of the many opportunities and complexities of the sport environment and the needs of competitive athletes should serve to enhance the psychological services available to competitive athletes. At the same time, increased knowledge of the context of competitive sport increases psychologists' understanding of the impact of culture on the individual.

REFERENCES

Andersen, M. B. (1996). Working with college student-athletes. In J. L. Van Raalte and B. W. Brewer (Eds.), *Exploring sport and exercise psychology.* Washington, DC: APA Books.

Andersen, M.B., Van Raalte, J. L., & Brewer, B. W. (1994). Assessing the skills of sport psychology supervisors. *The Sport Psychologist, 8,* 238-247.

Baillie, P. H. F., & Ogilvie, B. C. (1996). Working with elite athletes. In J. L. Van Raalte and B. W. Brewer (Eds.), *Exploring sport and exercise psychology.* Washington, DC: APA Books.

Brewer, B. W. (1993). Self-identity and specific vulnerability to depressed mood. *Journal of Personality, 61,* 343-364.

Brewer, B. W., Van Raalte, J. L., & Linder, D. E. (1993). Athletic identity: Hercules' muscles or achilles heel? *International Journal of Sport Psychology 24,* 237-254.

Gardner, F. (1995). The coach and the team psychologist: An integrated organizational model. In S. Murphy (Ed.), *Sport psychology interventions* (pp. 147-173). Champaign, IL: Human Kinetics.

Hale, B. D. (1995). Exclusive athletic identity: A predictor of positive or negative psychological characteristics? In R. Vanfraechem-Raway & Y. Vanden Auweele (Eds.) *IXth European Congress on Short Psychology: Proceedings* (pp. 466-472). Brussels, Belgium: Belgian Federation of Sport Psychology.

Hellstedt, J. C. (1995). Invisible players: A family systems mode. In S. Murphy (Ed.), *Sport psychology interventions* (pp. 117-146). Champaign, IL: Human Kinetics.

Linder, D. E., Brewer, B. W., Van Raalte, J. L., & DeLange, N. (1991). A negative halo for athletes who consult sport psychologists: Replication and extension. *Journal of Sport & Exercise Psychology, 13,* 133-148.

Pearson, R. E., & Petitpas, A. J. (1990). Transitions of athletes: Developmental and preventive perspectives. *Journal of Counseling & Development, 69,* 7-10.

Petitpas, A. J. (1978). Identity foreclosure: A unique challenge. *Personnel and Guidance Journal, 56,* 558-561.

Petitpas, A. J., & Champagne, D. E. (1988). Developmental programming for intercollegiate athletes. *Journal of College Student Development, 29,* 454-460.

Petrie, G. (1993). Injury from the athlete's point of view. In J. Heil (Ed.), *Psychology of sport injury* (pp. 17-23). Champaign, IL: Human Kinetics.

Taylor, J. & Schneider, B. A. (1992). The sport-clinical intake protocol: A comprehensive interviewing instrument for applied sport psychology. *Professional Psychology: Research and Practice, 23,* 318-325.

Van Raalte, J. L., Brewer, B. W., Brewer, D. D., & Linder, D. E. (1992). NCAA Division II college football players' perceptions of an athlete who consults a sport psychologist. *Journal of Sport & Exercise Psychology, 14,* 273-282.

Weinberg, R. S., & Gould, D. (1995). *Foundations of sport and exercise psychology.* Champaign, IL: Human Kinetics.

Insights into Effective
Sport Psychology Consulting

Daniel Gould
Nicole Damarjian

SUMMARY. This article discusses ways in which consultant characteristics and styles interact to influence intervention effectiveness in applied sport psychology. In particular, it is designed to provide therapists, counselors and psychologists with consulting guidelines that research and experience suggest are important for successfully implementing educationally-based mental skills training programs for athletes. Areas discussed include: (1) gaining entry and connecting with athletes; (2) identifying program objectives; (3) identifying specific strategies to achieve program objectives; (4) scheduling mental skills training; and (5) evaluating program effectiveness. It is emphasized that effective sport psychological consulting is a dynamic process including a collaborative relationship between the athlete, coach and sport psychologist. *[Article copies available for a fee from The Haworth Document Delivery Service: 1-800-342-9678. E-mail address: getinfo@haworth.com]*

INSIGHTS INTO EFFECTIVE
SPORT PSYCHOLOGY CONSULTING

Amy is a Division I collegiate basketball player. She frequently experiences high levels of stress during competition that inhibit her performance.

Daniel Gould, PhD, is affiliated with the Department of Exercise and Sport Science, University of North Carolina at Greensboro, Greensboro, NC 27412-5001 (E-mail: GOULDD.IRIS@UNCG.EDU).
Nicole Damarjian is affiliated with the University of North Carolina at Greensboro.

[Haworth co-indexing entry note]: "Insights into Effective Sport Psychology Consulting." Gould, Daniel, and Nicole Damarjian. Co-published simultaneously in *The Psychotherapy Patient* (The Haworth Press, Inc.) Vol. 10, No. 3/4, 1998, pp. 111-130; and: *Integrating Exercise, Sports, Movement and Mind: Therapeutic Unity* (ed: Kate F. Hays) The Haworth Press, Inc., 1998, pp. 111-130. Single or multiple copies of this article are available for a fee from The Haworth Document Delivery Service [1-800-342-9678, 9:00 a.m. - 5:00 p.m. (EST). E-mail address: getinfo@haworth.com].

111

Following the advice of her coach, she seeks help at the university counseling center. After several sessions, Amy has experienced little improvement and is skeptical as to the counselor's effectiveness. She questions the counselor's understanding of basketball and the unique demands that typically confront athletes. In addition, the counselor has failed to provide any practical suggestions for her to actually implement during practice and competition. Discouraged, Amy decides not to continue with counseling.

Jim is a clinical psychologist with a growing interest in the area of sport psychology. To explore this area further, he volunteers his services to a local high school baseball team. Although Jim is knowledgeable about baseball, he fails to gain the respect and support of some members of the coaching staff. As one assistant coach comments "sport psychology is for head-cases who are afraid to put in the physical training that is necessary to be great." Because of comments like this, those athletes who are curious about sport psychology are reluctant to express their interest to Jim. They fear being seen as a "head case" and being benched during a critical game or cut from the team.

Jan has won several major tennis titles. Unfortunately, recent marital problems have led to a state of serious depression and made it difficult for her to focus on her tennis. For several weeks she has been hitting the ball poorly and seriously considers withdrawing from the upcoming Australian Open. At her coach's request, she begins work with a sport psychologist. She is hesitant, however, to fully disclose her problems. Jan is concerned that the psychologist, a recreational tennis player and ardent fan, is eager to work with her primarily because of her celebrity status. Having been approached by many individuals in the past who wanted to be associated with her only because of her tennis accomplishments, Jan finds it difficult to completely trust the therapist.

What is it that has turned these and other athletes away from sport psychology and mental training? Considering the substantial research supporting the effectiveness of psychological interventions to enhance athletic performance and positively influence cognitive affective states, it is unlikely that psychological interventions are not effective. (See Burton, 1990; Greenspan & Feltz, 1989; Mace, 1990; Murphy, 1994; Vealey, 1994; and Weinberg, 1994 for comprehensive reviews.) However, it is unfortunate that most of this research has focused on whether general intervention techniques such as imagery, relaxation training, and goal setting are effective. There has been much less attention focused on *how* consultants can best implement these techniques. Similarly, only scant consideration has been given to how consultant characteristics and styles may influence intervention effectiveness.

Although a consultant may possess an adequate knowledge base and have extensive experience working in a more traditional clinical setting, several important issues need to be considered when working with athletes. For example, what consultant characteristics are athletes most responsive to? Amy might have been more inclined to remain in counseling if her counselor had made an effort to better understand the sport of basketball. That is, the counselor might have considered attending some games, learning more about the sport, and conferring with colleagues who have worked with basketball players, in an effort to understand the unique pressures placed on these athletes. Perhaps this would have allowed her counselor to provide Amy with more practical suggestions for practice and competition. Another concern when working with athletes involves strategies to promote coach support and follow-up. Jim might have received greater support from the baseball coaching staff had he first established a consultative relationship with the coaches. He might have been able to dispel common misconceptions surrounding sport psychology. Consultants and therapists must also recognize special considerations which must be contemplated when working with elite athletes, such as Jan, who are cautious of "outsiders" wanting to exploit their athletic success for their own benefit or notoriety. It is important to examine these and other issues in order to successfully work with coaches and athletes. After all, the effectiveness of any psychological intervention is dependent not only on the selection of an appropriate and reliable technique or set of techniques, but also the effective implementation of this intervention.

The purpose of this article is to provide therapists, counselors, and psychologists with consulting guidelines that research and experience suggest are important for successfully implementing a mental skills training program to meet the diverse needs of athletes. Mental skills training "refers to procedures that enhance an athlete's ability to use his or her mind effectively and readily in the execution of sport-related goals" (Gould & Damarjian, in press). The focus is not on treating clinical issues or psychotherapy. Rather, the emphasis is educational. In particular, strategies and techniques such as goal setting, anxiety management, relaxation training, and imagery are taught to normally functioning individuals. This is done in an effort to enhance athlete performance as well as psychological attributes such as self-confidence.

While the focus of this article is on mental skills training for normally functioning athletes, topics discussed may also be relevant to psychotherapists and clinicians working with athletes with clinical concerns such as Jan. Increasingly, recent research has shown that therapists who work in clinical settings with athletes have little background in sport psychology

(Petrie & Diehl, 1995). Hence, this article may help these individuals understand the unique sport context. The five areas to be discussed in this article include: (1) gaining entry and connecting with athletes; (2) identifying program objectives; (3) identifying specific strategies to achieve these objectives; (4) scheduling mental skills training; and (5) evaluating program effectiveness.

GAINING ENTRY AND CONNECTING WITH ATHLETES

Although each situation presents its own unique set of challenges, often one of the first issues to confront a sport psychologist involves gaining the respect and trust of coaches and athletes. Several barriers to entry have been identified by coaches, athletes, and consultants. These include: (1) the stereotypical "shrink" image; (2) lack of sport-specific knowledge; (3) inadequate knowledge of organizational politics and power structures; (4) failure to pay the necessary dues to earn the athletes' and coaches' respect; (5) sport "hero worship"; and (6) failure to be practical in an athletic environment. This section will address each of these consulting issues and will make specific suggestions as to how to handle potential problems.

Overcoming the Stereotypical "Shrink" Image

One of the most common misconceptions a sport psychology consultant implementing a mental skills intervention must overcome is the "shrink" image with which they are often associated (Ravizza, 1988). Therefore, effective consultants recognize that athletes respond much better to clinicians who they perceive do not act in a stereotypical "shrink" manner, while dispelling any stigmas they may have about individuals needing clinical assistance.

Many coaches and athletes assume that consultation with a sport psychologist implies clinical problems. Moreover, they do not have an accurate understanding of clinical psychology and instead have opinions based on inappropriate stereotypes conveyed in the entertainment media. Consequently, many athletes are apprehensive about working with a sport psychology consultant because they fear others, especially their coach, will assume they are a "head-case."

Given the above, it is critical that consultants explain initially what mental training is and is not. Consultants working with teams or in mental skills training educational settings should emphasize that most of their work is aimed at helping healthy normal functioning athletes maximize their potential on a more consistent basis. In the event that clinical issues, such as eating disorders or substance abuse, do arise, athletes need to understand that these are not personality flaws or signs of personal failure, but disorders which may afflict all types of individuals, including athletes.

Finally, in addition to doing the above, some consultants have found it effective to avoid the term psychologist (even if they are a licensed psychologist). Instead, they refer to themselves as performance enhancement specialists or mental trainers in an effort to avoid the "shrink" stereotype and the negative consequences associated with it.

Lack of Sport-Specific Knowledge

Another barrier to entry is a lack of sport-specific knowledge (Ravizza, 1988). It is difficult to gain the respect and credibility necessary to successfully implement a mental skills training program or intervention if a consultant is unable to speak the athletes' "language" or understand the task-relevant demands of their specific sport. For example, effective consultants realize the psychological demands for a contact sport such as football (e.g., fear of physical injury; large amounts of time devoted to game-film analysis) might differ significantly from a noncontact sport such as golf (e.g., where thought management is so critical because of the large amount of time not spent actually executing the skills of the game). Coaches and athletes will respond more favorably to a consultant who can design a mental skills training program around the specific needs of their sport, rather than a consultant who simply presents a generic prepackaged program (Orlick & Partington, 1987; Partington & Orlick, 1987).

Given the importance of demonstrating adequate knowledge of a particular sport, including an understanding of general terminology as well as basic strategies, what steps can consultants take to increase their sport knowledge? Prior to working with a sport, consultants can develop a knowledge base through reading, studying videos, taking physical education courses, or talking with people who participate in the sport. Another option is for consultants to actually participate in the sport themselves. For example, when working with the U.S. freestyle mogul ski team, the first author took several ski lessons in order to better understand certain aspects of skiing. While he never developed tremendous competence in the sport, he did develop a better appreciation of its demands. Finally, it is important that consultants acknowledge what they do not know rather than try to fake an understanding. For example, while failing to demonstrate sport-specific knowledge is a generally ineffective consulting practice, an even more ineffective practice is to unknowingly demonstrate incompetence by using terminology incorrectly or by failing to respect the intricacies of high-level sport. Coaches and athletes will appreciate a consultant who demonstrates a sincere interest and readiness to learn more about their sport (Partington & Orlick, 1987). Hence, when working with unfamiliar sports or in levels of the sport at which they have not competed (e.g., college basketball is much different from high school basketball), consultants must recognize the fact that they do not know as much as they would like, demonstrate their willingness to learn, and ask athletes and coaches to provide feedback if they make inappropriate applications in examples.

Inadequate Knowledge of Organizational Politics and Power Structures

A third barrier to entry is an inadequate knowledge of organizational politics and formal and informal structures of power. Coaches often make decisions regarding retention or release of a consultant partially on the basis of feedback from athletes and other staff members (Partington & Orlick, 1987). For instance, while working with a major college football team, a sport psychology consultant recognize the importance of the head athletic trainer's opinion of him and his services. Because the head trainer had been the head coach's trusted confidant for many years, he had even more influence than some members of the coaching staff in staffing decisions. Therefore, it is important that a consultant recognize the importance of gaining support at all levels of the organization, including assistant coaches, athletic trainers, physicians, and the equipment staff. If just one influential person misunderstands the consultant's role or intentions, the success of a mental skills training program is in jeopardy. It is also important that consultants educate the entire staff as to what sport psychology is as well as the role each individual can play to ensure the program's goals and objectives are met. Specifically, consultants should clearly define their role by discussing issues regarding confidentiality and team selection (Van Raalte, in press). Prior to consulting with individual athletes and teams, it is important to educate coaches about confidentiality issues. Consultants, athletes, coaches, and management should also discuss and establish clear expectations regarding the consultant's role in team selection and player retention.

Paying Your Dues

Gaining credibility and respect also requires patiently "paying your dues." Inexperienced consultants often have unrealistic expectations about the amount of time necessary to "connect" with an athlete or a team. They expect immediate rapport and dramatic results. Similarly, most athletes and coaches are not impressed by academic credentials or one's reputation as a psychologist. However, seasoned sport psychologists realize they must first gain credibility by demonstrating a sincere interest and genuine concern for the athletes they hope to work with. Often this requires a willingness to travel to various training camps. Athletes respond favorably to consultants who are available on a regular basis and are able to work with them individually (Orlick & Partington, 1987). Gaining credibility also requires attending practices and games despite inclement weather. Typically athletes gain respect for consultants they perceive to be "down-to-earth" and willing to get a little messy once in a while. Finally, paying your dues may require working for low salary until the consultant can demonstrate the value of his or her services.

Avoiding Sport "Hero-Worship"

When first establishing a relationship with elite athletes and coaches it is important to realize the time necessary to develop trust and rapport. Elite athletes and coaches are often skeptical of new people or "outsiders" (Hardy, Jones, & Gould, 1996). The story of Jan, the elite tennis player described at the beginning of this article, is not uncommon. Elite athletes, especially those with high visibility, are often approached by individuals who want to know them for their celebrity status or hope to use the athletes' celebrity status for their own benefit. Consultants in these situations must be especially patient. Inexperienced consultants often make the mistake of approaching a high-profile athlete too soon. For example, when first consulting with a professional team, it may be tempting to immediately provide mental training to the "star athlete." However, it is better for consultants to wait and let these athletes approach them after they have established that they are trustworthy and have something valuable to offer.

Finally, the athletic environment tends to be very informal and often times consultants are expected to socialize with coaches and athletes. This raises a number of questions about dual relationships. Consultants hoping to work in sport will find it helpful to reflect on the philosophical and ethical implications of such actions before they arise.

Use Concrete Terms and Be Practical

The final barrier to entry includes a failure to provide concrete, practical suggestions that are specific to the athletes' environment. When consultants are unable to effectively apply psychological principles to a specific sport, athletes rate consultants unsatisfactory and recommend not rehiring them (Orlick & Partington, 1987). As discussed earlier, this may include inadequate sport knowledge. Consultants must be able to speak the language of the sport as well as understand the relevant task demands. If consultants do not sufficiently understand the nature of the sport they are working with, it is unlikely they will be able to provide practical suggestions for the athletes to apply in training or competitive situations. For example, many therapists can teach athletes progressive relaxation. To be effective in sport settings, however, the therapist must also understand the demands of the particular sport in which the client takes part. Such factors as the optimal arousal level needed for best performance, the timing involved in performing a particular task, and the physical demand placed on the athlete must be understood. This will insure that the athlete does not become too relaxed.

Understanding the nature of the sport will also help the consultant teach the athlete to effectively incorporate the relaxation response into an actual game setting. For instance, a wrestler might use relaxation after going out of bounds or a baseball/softball pitcher might use relaxation on the mound after throwing a bad pitch. The key is to help the athlete find the most appropriate time to relax in the competitive setting.

Further, consultants must also be flexible in meeting the individual needs of the athletes they are working with, rather than imposing one method for all athletes in all sports. The same mental skills strategies are not equally effective with all athletes or for all psychological problems athletes confront.

Gaining entry and connecting with athletes requires that a consultant establish mutual respect, credibility, and trust with both coaches and athletes. Consultants need to be able to anticipate potential obstacles and develop the necessary strategies to effectively deal with these situations. Without this, it is unlikely that even the best mental skills training program will be effective.

Finally, it is important to recognize that not all consultants are right for every consulting situation. Despite doing everything "right," there are times when things simply do not work out. For example, the personality of the consultant may not match the personality of the coach or athlete. Organizational politics may dictate that effective consultants implementing quality programs are dropped due to "priority" shifts in the organization. Although these situations can be difficult to cope with, especially after committing time to a given program, consultants must accept these setbacks as part of the job.

IDENTIFYING PROGRAM OBJECTIVES

After understanding how to "connect" and establish credibility with coaches and athletes, it is time to determine specific objectives of the mental training program. As discussed earlier, athletes tend to respond more favorably to a program individualized to meet their and their sports' unique needs rather than a generic prepackaged program (Orlick & Partington, 1987). Assessing an athlete or team's strengths and weaknesses can include a variety of approaches. (See Heil and Henschen [1996] for a review of sport psychology assessments.) For example, a sport psychologist may choose to administer a standardized questionnaire such as the athletic coping skills inventory (Smith, Schutz, Smoll, & Pfacek, 1995), the Test of Attention and Interpersonal Style (Nideffer, 1990) or the Profile of Mood States (McNair, Lorr, & Dropplemann, 1971) to determine levels of key sport psychological variables in athletes (e.g., peaking under pressure, goal setting, mental preparation, concentration, tendency to become distracted and overloaded, ability to narrow attention, tension, vigor). However, sport psychologists are cautioned in the use of such inventories. Some athletes may not like these forms of assessment, especially if they are never given specific and practical feedback regarding their results (Orlick & Partington, 1987). Moreover, sport personality researchers (see Vealey [1992] for review) have clearly shown that many sport personality measures are inappropriate for use in team selection. An alternative approach might involve the Sport-Clinical Intake Protocol developed by Taylor and Schneider (1992). This would assist the clinician in screening for psychopathology that would merit more than mental training. In addition, the Group Environment Questionnaire may be used as a measure of group cohesion (Carron, Widmeyer, & Brawley, 1985). Overall, whether assessment includes a structured psychological test, a clinical intake form, informal interviews, and/or observation, the best method is the one with which the consultant and client feel most comfortable.

Recently, the application of performance profiling has been popularized to help sport psychologists and coaches identify areas of psychological strength and weakness as well as any discrepancies that may exist between coach and athlete perceptions of performance (Butler & Hardy, 1992; Butler, Smith, & Irwin, 1993). The basic method of performance profiling includes first eliciting from athletes what they perceive to be the fundamental psychological qualities of elite performance in their specific sport. For example, athletes typically cite psychological factors such as confidence, anxiety management, motivation, and commitment when doing the brainstorming portion of performance profiling. When facilitating this process, however, it is helpful if the sport psychology consultant is familiar with the psychological characteristics of successful athletes (Williams & Krane, 1993). Probing questions such as "What about imagery? Is that important for athletes in your sport?" help athletes derive performance profile areas.

After brainstorming a broad range of qualities and listing them as segments on a pie chart (see Figure 1), athletes are then asked to assess themselves along these constructs. For example, a golfer views concentration to be a key ingredient to success. She rates her own concentration

FIGURE 1. Performance Profile Example

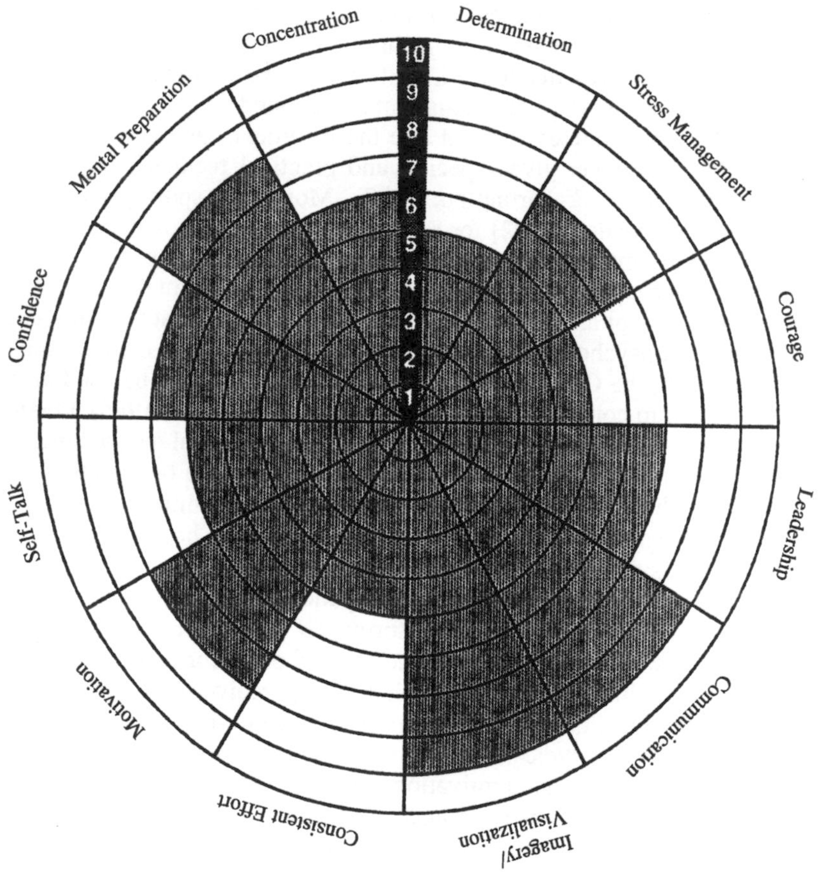

skills to be a 6 on a scale from 1 to 10, 1 representing low skill ability and 10 high skill ability. Having identified a discrepancy between current and desired skill levels, the golfer is then encouraged to establish appropriate goals with respect to those qualities that are most in need of change. For instance, the golfer may set a goal of increasing her concentration performance profile rating from 6 to 9 over the course of the summer. To do this the golfer will work with her consultant on concentration strategies such as the identification of specific task cues to focus on during critical moments of her round, thought stopping, and centered breathing. Moreover, the golfer is instructed to use these techniques during competitive simulations to ensure that she is able to effectively employ them under competitive conditions. After learning and implementing such techniques, goal progress is assessed by having the player rate concentration on the 1 to 10 scale after each tournament played.

Coaches may also be asked to assess individual athletes to determine whether or not their perceptions differ from those of the athlete (see Figure 2). It is important that both coaches and athletes agree on what areas need improvement to ensure a commitment to common goals and objectives. If they do not agree (as in the case example in Figure 2 regarding ratings on self-talk and mental preparation), the coach and athlete can discuss why they differ. Often this may reflect a difference in semantics or personal definitions of various psychological factors. However, on other occasions it reflects a difference of opinion between the two parties which must be recognized and addressed over time.

One benefit of performance profiling is that it empowers athletes to decide for themselves what areas of their performance require improvement. This is also likely to minimize problems related to adherence. Rather than assuming a relatively passive role, athletes are given the opportunity to actively shape the content of their training program, thereby enhancing feelings of ownership and intrinsic motivation. The pie chart also visually depicts or profiles their current psychological skills and attributes and provides a good starting point for an intervention. (For a more detailed review of the theory and application of performance profiling, the interested reader is directed to Butler, 1989; Butler & Hardy, 1992; Butler, Smith, & Irwin, 1993; and Jones, 1993.)

After assessing individual strengths and weaknesses, it is equally important to prioritize those skills that are most needed. For example, a swim coach may wish to help his or her athlete improve concentration, intrinsic motivation, confidence, and leadership skills. Some coaches are eager to try all that mental training has to offer. A consultant needs to help coaches select those skills and developmental sequences that are most

FIGURE 2. Coach-Athlete Performance Profile Comparison Example

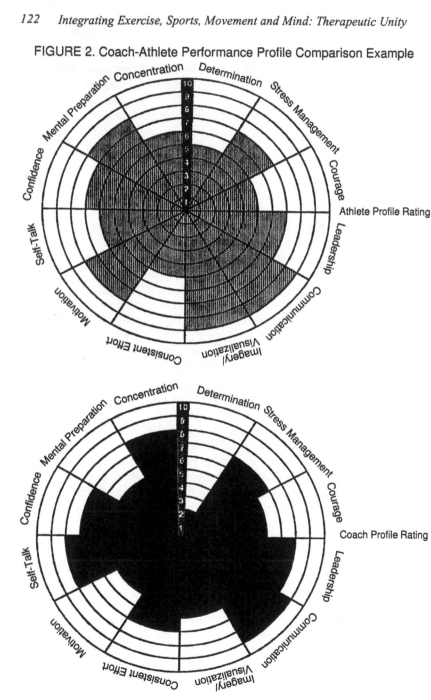

appropriate given the constraints of the individual situation. Such constraints may include how much time coaches and athletes are willing to devote to mental skills training as well as when during the season the program is to be implemented (Weinberg & Williams, 1993). If a coach is committed to implementing a mental training program over the course of an entire season, more skills can be introduced and developed over time. However, often a sport psychologist is asked to implement a program midseason when time is limited. Under these conditions, it would be unrealistic to attempt to develop more than one or two psychological skills. Generally, it is best that consultants help the athlete to develop a few well-learned skills that can be successfully employed. This will help create or maintain an interest in mental training in the future. If consultants try to do too much too soon, they risk accomplishing little as well as losing credibility and respect.

Finally, when establishing program objectives, consultants must be honest with coaches about what they can realistically expect from mental training, given the time and commitment they are willing to put forth. Mental skills will not make up for poor physical skills or techniques. Furthermore, like physical skills, mental skills require systematic practice. Consultants who promise dramatic performance improvements only set themselves up for failure and undermine the credibility of mental training (Ravizaa, 1988).

IDENTIFYING SPECIFIC STRATEGIES TO ACHIEVE OBJECTIVES

Once the sport psychologist, coach, and athlete agree on what psychological skills are in need of improvement, the next question is how best to achieve these desired changes. Sport psychologists must ask themselves, "What techniques or strategies will work best with this individual athlete or team given this situation or context?" Unfortunately, there are rarely simple or straightforward answers to this question. For example, a misinformed consultant may inaccurately assume everyone needs to incorporate visualization into their preperformance routines if they are to perform best. Research and practice suggest, however, that while more successful competitors have better delineated mental preparation routines and often use imagery, not all routines involve imagery (Gould, Ekiund & Jackson, 1992). These routines tend to be highly individualized. Incorporating imagery into a preperformance routine for one athlete may be highly effective and desirable; however, doing so for a second athlete may have negative effects.

It is critical for psychologists and therapists with little formal sport psychology training to take time to review the sport-specific research and literature to better ensure choosing the most appropriate intervention strategy. Applied sport psychology has a long and rich history dating back to the early 1900s and the work of Coleman Griffith at the University of Illinois (Griffith, 1925). The field has continued to grow, culminating in tremendous consulting interest over the last 15 years. Therefore, if the most appropriate mental skills training strategies are to be selected, a solid understanding of this body of knowledge is needed. Recommended readings include Burton's (1992) and Gould's (1993) reviews of goal setting; Murphy and Jowdy's (1992) and Vealey and Walter's (1993) reviews of mental rehearsal imagery; Bunker, Williams, and Zinsser's (1993) review of self-talk; and Gould and Udry's (1994) review of relaxation and arousal regulation strategies. Comprehensive textbooks in the area include Weinberg and Gould's (1995) *Foundations of Sport and Exercise Psychology,* Van Raalte and Brewer's (1996) *Exploring Sport and Exercise Psychology,* and Williams's (1993) *Applied Sport Psychology.*

MENTAL SKILLS TRAINING SCHEDULE

After identifying the most appropriate intervention strategy, it is important to determine a mental skills training schedule. One issue to consider is the timing for implementation of a mental skills training program. Ideally, it is best to introduce a mental skills training program during the off-season or early in preseason (Martens, 1987; Weinberg & Williams, 1993). Coaches at this point typically have fewer demands on their time and therefore are better able to help plan and deliver a training program. It is also a time when athletes can practice various psychological techniques without the immediate pressure of competition.

Unfortunately, many coaches turn to mental training mid-season in a panic to revive their team after a series of poor performances. This may be the worst time to implement a mental skills training program, not only because of the extra demands on both coaches and athletes, but also because mental skills, like physical skills, require practice before they can be mastered.

Despite the logic of focusing on mental skills training in the pre- or off-season, coaches and athletes may be less motivated during these times. Hence, while it is best to start mental skills training in the off-season or preseason, it is not always possible to do so. Consultants should not be overly concerned if they must begin their efforts at other times of the season as many successful efforts have been carried out in non-optimal times of the year. Consultants must be cognizant, however, that in the off-season some athletes must be "sold" on sport psychology before they are motivated to practice mental skills.

This leads to the question of how long a mental skills training program should last. Ideally, mental skills training should become an integral part of daily practice. Mental skills, like physical skills, require systematic practice to develop and maintain at a given level of proficiency. Unfortunately, some athletes mistakenly assume mental training does not work, when in fact they have not practiced sufficiently to warrant a noticeable change in performance, especially under the pressures of competition.

This is not to suggest that mental skills take precedence over physical skills. Both are important components of performance success. Moreover, it is not always necessary to isolate mental from physical skill training. Integrating mental training into daily practice not only fosters a commitment to the development of mental skills, but also has other potential benefits. Some of these include the acquisition of physical skills by helping athletes clarify practice objectives, focus on the most relevant skills needing practice, facilitate the formulation of motor plans, effectively process performance feedback, and assist in the refinement of motor programs (Sinclair & Sinclair, 1994).

Unfortunately, sport psychologists are rarely able to meet with a team or athlete on a daily basis. Therefore, it is critical that coaches reinforce mental training in the consultant's absence. Coaches have considerable power over athletes (Van Raalte, in press). Sport psychologists, then, can be of great help to coaches by outlining specific ways to integrate mental skills training into practice. For example, during instruction, a coach may suggest athletes take 5 seconds to imagine a correct performance in their mind following a mistake. Similarly, following a successful performance, athletes may be encouraged to take a few moments to recognize and reinforce what they did well. It is important to remind coaches that integrating mental and physical skill training does not necessarily imply disrupting practice for 10 minutes to discuss mental skills. Finally, the consultant often serves as a mental skills training resource for the coach. It is therefore important that the consultant be familiar with the literature on the psychology of coaching (Martens, 1987).

It is essential that sport psychologists find ways to maintain coach support throughout the season (Ravizza, 1988; Weinberg & Williams, 1993). At the start of a season, many coaches are enthusiastic about implementing a mental skills training program. Unfortunately, as the season progresses and coaches have greater time demands and pressures, mental training may be reduced to a handful of brief meetings added on to an already demanding practice schedule. Coach involvement in mental skills training and follow-up on a daily basis is essential to program success. Athletes will be more likely to commit to a mental skills training program when their coaches designate quality practice time to it. Hence, one way to increase program effectiveness is for sport psychologists to form working partnerships with coaches, both supplementing their efforts at mental skills training and facilitating their awareness of continued emphasis and involvement.

PROGRAM EVALUATION

The final step in any successful mental training program involves evaluating whether or not the program is meeting its established objectives (Weinberg & Williams, 1993). For example, assume a consultant has designed a goal setting program for a local high school basketball team. The week before official practice begins, the consultant meets with the team to introduce mental skills training and the importance of goal setting. With the help of the coach, he or she identifies several team goals such as arriving on time for practice each day and qualifying for the state championship. The consultant also meets with several athletes to determine specific individual goals. As the season progresses the consultant evaluates the effectiveness of the goal setting program to determine what, if any, progress has been made. Are practices more efficient and productive? How are players progressing with regard to their individual goals? For those athletes who have shown little improvement, individual meetings are set up to identify possible problems. Depending on the situation, the coach may need to identify a different practice strategy to help the athlete achieve his or her goals. Those athletes that are improving are encouraged to continue with goal setting.

Effective consultants vary widely in the degree of formality of their evaluations (Hardy, Jones, & Gould, 1996). Although evaluations may include more formal questionnaires or inventories, often evaluations take the form of subjective and informal discussion with the performer and the coach. For example, when consulting with the United States freestyle mogul ski team, the first author evaluated the effectiveness of their mental skills training program in several ways. One was to examine individual and team performances. How did the athletes finish in the World Cup Championship and what were their performance rankings relative to the other top skiers in the world? A second form of evaluation involved subjective feedback received from coaches and athletes regarding what effect, if any, they felt the program had on performance. This type of feedback was deemed especially helpful because many non-psychological factors influence elite skier performance (e.g., weather, equipment, physical conditioning, injury). Performance standings and rankings can at times be misleading. Subjective evaluations, however, allow the coaches and athletes to factor in such variables in their assessments of program effectiveness.

Program evaluations provide important feedback as to what strategies are effective and for whom they are effective. If the program is meeting its objectives, the sport psychologist can continue with confidence. However, if the program is not meeting its objectives, it is critical to determine why. What obstacles are preventing the program's success and what strategies can be employed to overcome these obstacles? Several common problems have already been discussed (e.g., establishing rapport with athletes and coaches, dispelling mental training myths). It is important to be aware of these potential problems and identify strategies to avoid or rectify them.

CONCLUSION

There are many ways to effectively implement a mental skills training program. Consulting with athletes, as with any other client population, is a dynamic process. It brings together in a collaborative relationship the efforts of several individuals including the athlete, sport psychologist, and coaching staff in pursuit of both athletic and personal excellence.

Although there are many effective ways to implement a mental skills training program and consult with athletes, several guidelines were suggested to help therapists and psychologists meet the diverse needs of athletes. These include: (1) gaining entry and connecting with athletes; (2) identifying program objectives; (3) identifying specific strategies to achieve these objectives; (4) scheduling mental skills training; and (5) evaluating program effectiveness. Integrating specific suggestions from each of these areas with a consultant's own personality and experience will serve to maximize a consultant's effectiveness.

REFERENCES

Bunker, L., Williams, J. M., & Zinsser, N. (1993). Cognitive techniques for improving performance and self-confidence. In J. M. Williams (Ed.) *Applied sport psychology: Personal growth to peak performance* (2nd ed., pp. 225-242). Palo Alto, CA: Mayfield

Burton, D. (1990). Multimodal stress management in sport: Current status and future directions. In J. G. Jones & L. Hardy (Eds.) *Stress and performance in sport* (pp. 171-202). Chichester: John Wiley & Sons.

Burton, D. (1992). The Jekyll/Hyde nature of goals: Reconceptualizing goal setting. In T. Horn (Ed.) *Advances in sport psychology* (pp. 267-297). Champaign, IL: Human Kinetics.

Butler, R. J. (1989). Psychological preparation of Olympic boxers. In J. Kremer & W. Crawford (Eds.) *The psychology of sport: Theory and practice* (pp. 78-84). Leicester, England: British Psychological Association.

Butler, R. J., & Hardy, L. (1992). The performance profile: Theory and application. *The Sport Psychologist, 6,* 253-264.

Butler, R. J., Smith, M., & Irwin, I. (1993). The performance profile in practice. *Journal of Applied Sport Psychology, 5,* 48-63.

Carron, A. V., Widmeyer, W. N., & Brawley, L. R. (1985). The development of an instrument to assess cohesion in sport teams: The Group Environmental Questionnaire. *Journal of Sport Psychology, 7,* 244-266.

Gould, D. (1993). Goal setting for peak performance. In J. Williams (Ed.) *Applied sport psychology: Personal growth to peak performance* (2nd ed., pp. 158-169). Palo Alto, CA: Mayfield.

Gould, D., & Damarjian, N. (in press). Mental skills training in sport. In B. C. Elliot (Ed.) Applied sport science: Training in sport. *International handbook of sport sciences*-Vol. 3. Sussex, England: John Wiley & Sons.

Gould, D., Eklund, R., & Jackson, S. (1992). 1988 US Olympic wrestling excellence: I. Mental preparation, precompetitive cognition, and affect. *The Sport Psychologist, 6,* 358-382.

Gould, D., & Udry, E. (1994). Psychological skills for enhancing performance: Arousal regulation strategies. *Medicine and Science in Sports and Exercise, 26,* 478-485.

Greenspan, M., & Feltz, D. (1989). Psychological interventions with athletes in competitive situations. *Journal of Sport Psychology 3,* 219-236.

Griffith, C. R. (1925). Psychology and its relation to athletic competition. *American Physical Education Review, 30,* 193-199.

Hardy, L., Jones, G., & Gould, D. (1996). *The psychological preparation of elite sports performers.* Chichester, United Kingdom: Wiley.

Heil, J., & Henschen, K. (1996). Assessment in sport and exercise psychology. In J. L. Van Raalte & B. W. Brewer (Eds.) *Exploring sport and exercise psychology* (pp. 229-255). Washington, DC: American Psychological Association.

Jones, J.G. (1993). The role of performance profiling in cognitive behavioral in sport. *The Sport Psychologist, 7,* 160-172.

Mace, R. (1990). Cognitive behavioral interventions in sport. In G. Jones & L. Hardy (Eds.) *Stress and performance in sport* (pp. 203-231). Chichester: John Wiley & Sons.

Martens, R. (1987). *Coaches guide to sport psychology.* Champaign, IL: Human Kinetics.

McNair, D. N., Lorr, M., & Droppleman, L.F. (1971). *Profile of mood states.* San Diego, CA: Education and Industrial Testing Service.

Murphy, S. M. (1994). Imagery interventions in sport. *Medicine and Science in Sports and Exercise 26,* 486-494.

Murphy, S. M., & Jowdy, D. (1992). Imagery and mental practice. In T. Horn (Ed.) *Advances in sport psychology* (pp. 221-250). Champaign, IL: Human Kinetics.

Nideffer, R. (1990). Using the test of attention and interpersonal style with elite athletes. In J. Bond, & J. Gross (Eds.). *Australian sport psychology: The eighties* (pp. 149-160). Canberra, Australia: Australian Institute of Sport.

Orlick, T., & Partington, J. (1987). The sport psychology consultant: Analysis of critical components as viewed by Canadian athletes. *The Sport Psychologist, 1,* 4-7.

Partington, J., & Orlick, T. (1987). The sport psychology consultant: Olympic coaches' views. *The Sport Psychologist, 1,* 95-102.

Petrie, T., & Diehl, N. (1995). Sport psychology in the profession of psychology. *Professional Psychology: Research and Practice. 26, 288-289.*

Ravizza, K. (1988). Gaining entry with athletic personnel for season-long consulting. *The Sport Psychologist 2(3)* 243-254.

Sinclair, G., & Sinclair, D. (1994). Developing reflective performers by integrating mental management skills with the learning process. *The Sport Psychologist,* 13-27.

Smith, R. E., Schutz, R. W., Smoll, F. L., & Pfacek, J. T. (1995). Development and validation of a multidimensional measure of sport-specific psychological skills: The athletic coping skills inventory-28. *Journal of Sport and Exercise Psychologist, 17,* 379-398.

Taylor, J., & Schneider, M. (1992). The sport-clinical intake protocol: A comprehensive intervention instrument for applied sport psychology. *Professional Psychology: Research and Practice, 23,* 318-325..

Van Raalte, J. L. (in press). The competitive athlete. *The Psychotherapy Patient, 10(3/4),* 101-110.

Van Raalte, J. L., & Brewer, B. W. (Eds.) *Exploring sport and exercise psychology* (pp. 229-255). Washington, DC: American Psychological Association.

Vealey, R. S. (1992). Personality in sport: A comprehensive review. In T. S. Horn (Ed.) *Advances in sport psychology* (pp. 25-59). Champaign, IL: Human Kinetics.

Vealey, R. S. (1994). Current status and prominent issues in sport psychology interventions. *Medicine and Science in Sports and Exercise, 26,* 495-502.

Vealey, R. S., & Walter, S. M. (1993). Imagery training for performance enhancement and personal growth. In J. Williams (Ed.) *Applied sport psychology: Personal growth to peak performance* (2nd ed., pp. 200-224). Palo Alto, CA: Mayfield.

Weinberg, R. S. (1994). Goal setting and performance in sport and exercise settings: A synthesis and critique. *Medicine and Science in Sports and Exercise, 26,* 469-477.

Weinberg, R. S., & Gould, D. (1995). *Foundations of sport and exercise psychology.* Champaign, IL: Human Kinetics.

Weinberg, R. S., & Williams, J. M. (1993). Integrating and implementing a psychological skills training program. In J. M. Williams (Ed.). *Applied sport psychology: Personal growth to peak performance* (2nd ed., pp. 274-298). Mountain View, CA: Mayfield Publishing Company.

Williams J. M. (Ed.) (1993). *Applied sport psychology: Personal growth to peak performance* (2nd ed.). Mountain View, CA: Mayfield Publishing Company.

Williams, J. M., & Wane, V. (1993). Psychological characteristics of peak performance. In J. M. Williams (Ed.). *Applied sport psychology: Personal growth to peak performance* (2nd ed., pp. 137-147). Mountain View, CA: Mayfield Publishing Company.

CLIENT VOICES

Putting the "Clinical" into Sport Psychology Consulting

Karen D. Cogan

SUMMARY. This article focuses on the clinical issues in a sport psychology consulting case. The client was a male wrestler who presented with concerns about depression due to retirement from his sport and the ending of a romantic relationship. The author discusses her role as a sport psychologist in allowing the athlete to explore and resolve his feelings about retirement. In addition, the evolving personal issues that surfaced throughout the therapeutic relationship are described. Conclusions about integrating personal and athletic concerns in sport psychology consulting are offered. *[Article copies available for a fee from The Haworth Document Delivery Service: 1-800-342-9678. E-mail address: getinfo@haworth.com]*

To many professionals and students in sport psychology, the term "sport psychology consulting" tends to evoke images of a consultant

Karen D. Cogan, PhD, is affiliated with the University of North Texas, Counseling and Testing Center, P.O. Box 13487, Denton, TX 76203 (E-mail: cogan@dsa.unt.edu).

[Haworth co-indexing entry note]: "Putting the 'Clinical' into Sport Psychology Consulting." Cogan, Karen D. Co-published simultaneously in *The Psychotherapy Patient* (The Haworth Press, Inc.) Vol. 10, No. 3/4, 1998, pp. 131-143; and: *Integrating Exercise, Sports, Movement and Mind: Therapeutic Unity* (ed: Kate F. Hays) The Haworth Press, Inc., 1998, pp. 131-143. Single or multiple copies of this article are available for a fee from The Haworth Document Delivery Service [1-800-342-9678, 9:00 a.m. - 5:00 p.m. (EST). E-mail address: getinfo@haworth.com].

131

conducting performance enhancement interventions, such as imagery, arousal regulation, and goal setting with athletes and/or teams. This image is fairly accurate as these interventions comprise much of what sport psychology consultants do. These interventions are more visible and often are demonstrated in continuing education workshops or at conferences (e.g., Ravizza, 1994; Taylor, McCann, & Horsely, 1994). Less information is available on how to work with an athlete who is struggling with a long-term "clinical" issue (e.g., depression, eating disorder). In fact, many psychologists working in clinical settings with individual athletes or teams have had little sport psychology training (Petrie & Diehl, 1995; Petrie, Diehl, & Watkins, 1995). With my "hybrid" training, which is grounded in both psychology and sport science, I have had the opportunity to blend my skills and examine clinical issues rather than focus exclusively on performance enhancement. Therefore, this article will focus on a long-term clinical therapy case with an athlete.

In many cases athletic performance difficulties do not occur in a vacuum. Improving concentration or managing anxiety may be the presenting issue, yet other life issues often are involved with a performance decrement and may even become the central concern (Van Raalte & Andersen, 1996). In general, athletic and personal issues interact, and I am able to address both while maintaining continuity in the therapeutic relationship. When an athlete approaches me for assistance, I assess his/her stated needs, and, through taking a history, determine what mix of athletic and personal concerns exist (Taylor & Schneider, 1992). Consequently, we work together to determine which issues to address and goals of therapy and/or consultation.

The following case outlines a 21-month therapeutic relationship with an athlete-client whom I will call Ryan. Ryan gave his permission to be the focus of this article; however, some information has been altered to preserve his anonymity. Even with some changes, this case exemplifies my clinical work with athletes.

EVALUATION

Referral

Ryan, a 24-year-old Caucasian former collegiate wrestler, began therapy with me to obtain a second opinion. A previous therapist and psychiatrist had diagnosed him with a thought disorder after conducting a clinical interview and administering a WAIS-R, Rorschach, TAT, and projective drawings. Ryan questioned this diagnosis and the validity of the testing.

He suspected that he was depressed, and that these non-athletically trained (Ryan labeled them "civilian") mental health professionals were not qualified to diagnose him without an understanding of his sport context. He found another psychiatrist who diagnosed him with Major Depressive Disorder and prescribed Prozac. Ryan then was referred to me, because of my identity as a sport psychology consultant, by a therapist whom he had consulted during his wrestling career. He specifically requested someone with sport psychology training as he previously had worked with a sport psychologist and did not want to experience any further misunderstandings with "civilian" psychologists.

Family History

Ryan's parents divorced when he was in seventh grade. He initially lived with his mother for a few years and later moved to his father's home where he remained throughout high school. He was confused about how the divorce occurred. He never received adequate explanations or help in coping with his emotional reactions to the upheaval in family relationships. In retrospect, he realized that he was uncertain about how he felt and wished his parents had been more active in asking him how he was coping and generally helping him through his confusion. In general, he learned to keep any feelings hidden, even from himself, and only through therapy realized that this event had been traumatic for him.

After the divorce, Ryan and his father developed a primarily financial relationship. His father insisted on supporting him financially, and their communications most often involved money. When Ryan approached his father with more personal issues, such as retiring from wrestling, his father did not listen well and typically had his own agenda for Ryan. Having been a competitive gymnast, his father pushed Ryan to persist and fight in the face of discomfort. These responses effectively eliminated Ryan's motivation to express emotional discontent in his father's presence. Ryan's father had remarried, and although Ryan reported having a good relationship with his step-mother, he still experienced some emotional distance from her as well.

Ryan felt very removed from his biological mother who lived in a different state. Her life was the complete opposite of what Ryan had envisioned for himself, and he did not relate to her or understand her. She smoked, was overweight, and worked at a low pay/low status job. In short, she was all the things that Ryan had never wanted to be, and he felt ambivalent about having a relationship with her. On one hand, he felt obligated to call and talk to her as her son; on the other hand, he felt so uncomfortable interacting with her that he avoided phone conversations for weeks at a time.

Ryan had one sister who was five years older than he. He described her as manipulative, especially in obtaining financial support from their father or any type of assistance from Ryan. She abused alcohol and drugs and was involved in extremely unstable dating relationships. Ryan was angry with her for her irresponsible behaviors, particularly because he valued his own characteristics of hard work and achievement, and felt little affiliation with her. He wanted to set limits with her, but the rest of the family continued to be blind to her behaviors and were unsupportive of his efforts.

Intake Information

Ryan presented with clear symptoms of major depression, including sadness, decreased appetite, decreased pleasure and interest in activities, excessive guilt, low energy, and decreased concentration. Ryan attributed his depression to two major issues: (1) lingering uncertainty about his decision (approximately three years prior to treatment with me) to retire from wrestling before his eligibility ended, and (2) the recent breakup with a girlfriend.

Wrestling. When Ryan began wrestling, he had always approached his training with intense determination and persistence. As he progressed, he evidenced substantial natural wrestling talent and was expected to perform well at the national level. Somewhere in all his preparation, however, Ryan lost the intrinsic motivation to become the best, and training became a chore. He questioned the choice of putting his body through the intense training and diet regimen required of wrestlers. When he tried discussing the option of retirement, his father encouraged him to persist and did not recognize Ryan's need to end his athletic career. Consequently, Ryan attempted to ignore any negative emotions, continued to wrestle, and felt "miserable" during that time. Finally, he decided to retire but felt guilty about giving up on a natural talent and could not forgive himself for being a "quitter." Even three years later, as he discussed his retirement with me, he expressed significant ambivalence and sadness about losing this part of his identity.

Ryan's reactions to retirement are similar to those documented in the sport psychology literature. Although some of the literature suggests that the majority of athletes are able to adjust to this transition (Greendorfer & Blinde, 1985), other studies report trauma and grief reactions (Blinde & Stratta, 1992; Hallinan & Snyder, 1987), sometimes for 10 years after retirement (Baillie, 1993). Retirement is viewed as a transition in an athlete's life that is influenced by many factors (Danish, Petitpas & Hale, 1992, 1993). One factor is the context of retirement; adverse reactions occur when disengagement from sport is involuntary. Although Ryan made a conscious choice to stop wrestling, a part of him was not ready to terminate his participation, and that part of him perceived his retirement as involuntary. Another factor influencing reactions to retirement is identification with the sport. Ogilvie and Howe (1986) discuss the identity crisis many athletes experience upon retiring as they give up a role that has been central to their lives. In Ryan's case, all of his identity was connected to wrestling, and retirement meant losing this important sense of self.

Relationship Concerns. Ryan dated frequently throughout adolescence and young adulthood; however, he never felt much emotional connection with the young women he dated. Serious, emotionally involved relationships were discouraged in wrestling due to the potential distraction from training. After retiring, Ryan developed a relationship that provided a stronger emotional connection, and felt sad and depressed when the relationship ended. He was trying to decide whether to pursue this relationship with the type of determination he utilized in wrestling training or to allow himself to heal from this second loss as well.

Diagnostic Impressions and Clinical Interpretations

I concurred with the second psychiatrist that Ryan was experiencing a major depressive episode. In addition, Ryan displayed other clinically interesting reactions. If he felt overwhelmed by emotion, he shifted into "brain cloud" mode which appeared to be a form of dissociation. From the time he was a child, but especially when he began facing the decision to stop wrestling, he utilized "brain cloud" mode as a coping mechanism. I suspect that as Ryan was coping with strong feelings related to wrestling, he periodically slipped into "brain cloud" so that he could continue training even in the face of adversity. Such persistence is admirable, but it also prevented him from retiring when he really wanted to do so. I also suspect that he was experiencing "brain cloud" during his interviews and testing with the former therapist, who interpreted this behavior as a thought disorder. The goals of therapy related to this issue were to assist Ryan in being more immediate and open with affect and help him identify the true emotions behind "brain cloud."

TREATMENT

Treatment focused on a variety of issues, some of which related to the history presented above and others that arose during the course of therapy.

In general, Ryan had difficulty identifying and expressing emotions, especially sadness and anger. Throughout his life, he had avoided painful affect and identified any negative feeling he experienced as stress or anxiety. In addition, Ryan had always been taught to suppress anger because anger in competition might cause him to lose focus.

Initially, Ryan wanted to examine his previous therapy experiences. I obtained psychological testing results from Ryan's former therapist in order to evaluate his mental functioning. Although some of the results might be interpreted as suggestive of a thought disorder, a thorough integration of all available information was more indicative of major depression. We processed Ryan's anger regarding the misdiagnosis and discussed strategies for resolution, such as discussing his feelings with the therapist or writing a letter. Ryan later confronted the therapist in person and continued to vent his anger and frustrations in sessions with me. Anger was not a familiar emotion for Ryan, and this issue was a critical point in therapy as he began to access this emotion. He challenged himself to experience and express anger in a productive and appropriate manner. This work allowed him to have easier access to subsequent emotions related to other issues in his life.

The first sessions also involved an exploration of Ryan's depression. We examined grief/loss issues related to his retirement from wrestling and the breakup with his girlfriend. He was extremely ambivalent about his decision to stop wrestling. Despite three years of reviewing this choice with various therapists, it continued to be a central concern. He could not give himself permission to have made such a choice and considered it a mistake to have given up his talent. He also struggled with the loss of his athlete identity because now he was more like the "civilians" he had avoided. He was walking the line between the athlete and non-athlete worlds and did not fit in either place. Just when he had convinced himself that retiring was a mistake, he recounted months of "misery" when he continued to train.

With my sport psychology training and my own athletic retirement experience, I easily understood his connection to the sport world and his prolonged emotional reactions to severing those ties. I knew the type of focused training he had lived because I had lived it also. Although many psychologists avoid self-disclosures, it was useful for me to briefly disclose some of my similar experiences related to training and retirement. This openness enhanced our rapport and allowed Ryan to view me differently than the previous therapist. I was able to communicate my understanding of his struggle and be patient while he worked toward permitting himself to have made the choice to retire.

Ryan felt a similar ambivalence regarding the breakup of his dating relationship. He vacillated between recognizing the dysfunctional dynamics (i.e., she was controlling and could be verbally abusive) that evolved and wanting to make the relationship work. Again, Ryan made important strides in the still unfamiliar affective realm when he allowed himself to experience intense grief and pain and tearfully examine these losses. In addition, Ryan began to achieve insight into the connection between these unresolved losses and the resulting depression. As therapy progressed, thoughts and emotions related to these two losses periodically reemerged, but each time Ryan was able to feel more deeply and accept his decisions regarding both issues.

Therapy then moved towards an examination of Ryan's relationships with his family of origin. He could most easily access feelings, primarily anger, towards his sister. He began to recognize that he did not like her and was not willing to be in a relationship with her if she continued to be manipulative. He began setting appropriate limits with her but became frustrated by his parents' inability to stop "enabling" her. For instance, each time she was in a car accident his father would buy her a new car, while Ryan's mother would call and plead with him to "be nice" to his sister when he was attempting to set limits. Ryan finally concluded that for his own sanity he would maintain a distance from her; he remained firm in this decision.

Accessing feelings about each of his parents and their divorce was more challenging. Ryan initially minimized the effects of his parents' divorce on him as well as the problems in his relationships with each parent. Rather than examine the effects of these experiences on his feelings and current emotional state, he wanted explanations and evidence to understand how these issues related to his depression. At first, Ryan could not articulate the issues surrounding the divorce. As therapy progressed, however, he began to recognize that his parents never explained the divorce to him and never helped him understand how it affected him. As a child he had been bewildered by the divorce and the chaos it created; he had no framework for expressing his feelings. Thus, he ignored his feelings and withdrew. The most painful component of his emotional reaction was that his parents were oblivious to the effects of their divorce on their son. He felt they never even *tried* to help him cope with his reactions. Gradually he began to see that avoiding these painful issues throughout his earlier life influenced his current mood.

Ryan also began to recognize issues related to growing up with an emotionally inexpressive and financially controlling father. Throughout therapy, Ryan worked on being more direct and honest with his father but continued to hold back some of his true feelings, such as anger and frustration. We role played conversations in which Ryan could express his true (and painful) feelings about his wrestling experience or his father's lack of awareness during the divorce. After Ryan became aware of the financial control his father exerted, he began individuating from his father by becoming more financially independent and preparing to eventually support himself.

Ryan struggled with defining the extent to which he wanted a relationship with his mother. He did not enjoy talking to her or spending time with her, yet felt guilty for not wanting much contact. Some very strong feelings of guilt and sadness were associated with this relationship, but he experienced a "block" when trying to examine feelings about her. At the time therapy terminated, due to his intent to pursue graduate school in another state, we had not adequately addressed his feelings about his mother. He continued to experience "brain cloud" when we discussed her and had difficulty accessing any emotion related to her.

Ryan substantially worked through the sadness he felt over the loss of his dating relationship. He gradually developed a realistic assessment of the difficulties in the relationship and let go of hope for reconciliation. He became involved in another relationship during the course of therapy. Ryan reported that the relationship with this woman was characterized by openness, honesty, and comfort; however, he did not experience the same attachment that he had felt in the previous relationship. He was satisfied in this relationship, but did not appear overly concerned when his plans to attend graduate school took him out of state and away from the relationship.

Another focus of therapy was eating and weight concerns. Wrestlers engage in a variety of pathogenic weight control behaviors to qualify for designated weight classifications. Each strives to wrestle in the lowest possible weight class because at the upper range of that class he presumably has an advantage in strength, speed, and leverage over his opponent (Brownell, Steen, & Wilmore, 1987). Typically wrestlers will fast and dehydrate themselves (e.g., by jogging in plastic sweatsuits or sitting in saunas) for weeks before, and especially just prior to, weigh-ins for competition (Nitzke, Voichick, & Olson, 1992). Unlike many non-sport eating disorders, wrestling weight control behaviors are not secretive. Athletes may discuss strategies to "make weight" and engage in these strategies together (Burches-Miller & Black, 1991). Also, the motivations for making weight are externally imposed by competition regulations and wrestlers may not view competition weight as ideal during the off-season.

Therefore, upon retirement sometimes wrestlers can transition to more "normal" eating patterns and views of weight.

We briefly discussed eating issues and body image concerns related to Ryan's career as a wrestler. Ryan repeatedly mentioned his erratic and restrictive eating behaviors and his self-induced deprivation. He commented that he had become so thirsty in the past that he would have been willing to drink muddy water off of the street if he thought it would not add weight. Even after retirement, he continued to restrict himself, although not to the degree he had for competition. He was disappointed that he had allowed himself to gain weight since retiring from wrestling and felt "fat." As an objective observer, I saw a thin and defined athletic physique, but he only saw how different he was from his wrestling days. His transition to "civilian" eating patterns had been difficult for him and was still in process. Although I confronted him on the need to examine body image and the issues underneath his eating behaviors, he was unwilling to delve too deeply into this area. I was comfortable with his choice because of my view that eating difficulties relate more to unexpressed emotions and unrealistic expectations about body appearance than food per se. Therefore, I continued to direct the focus towards emotional exploration and reducing his need for perfection.

Finally, we addressed his questions and concerns about career goals and the possibility of graduate school in clinical psychology. During the last months of therapy, a portion of many sessions was devoted to coping with the stress of the application process. When we terminated therapy, he was preparing to move to another state and attend a university as a non-degree graduate student. He intended to work towards being admitted into a graduate program at that university.

Process Issues in Therapy

Rapport was enhanced initially by my own experience as a collegiate gymnast. As previously mentioned, Ryan was quick to distinguish between athletes who knew and had experienced the sport culture and "civilians" who could never really understand. In addition, my training in sport psychology and certification as a sport psychology consultant made Ryan feel more comfortable with my credentials. Although it is not necessary for one to have competitive athletic experiences to be a successful sport psychology consultant (Danish, Petitpas, & Hale, 1993), in this case it was clear that my athletic background, coupled with my educational experiences, was essential to begin our work together. Ryan commented that it was easier to immediately begin working rather than initially focus on educating his therapist about his sport experience. He felt more comfortable because he did not have to explain his "athlete world view" and could talk the language without having to define terminology for me. Also, after previously experiencing a negative therapeutic relationship, Ryan was looking for someone who was credible and knowledgeable about his "culture" and issues.

A second process issue involved an exploration of our therapeutic relationship. Ryan had been taking undergraduate courses in counseling as he prepared for graduate school and began learning about the importance of strong therapeutic relationships. Early in therapy we began discussing how we were working together and our impressions of each other. Ryan confronted me on my responses to him in some instances and discussed his periodic discomfort in therapy. For example, he wanted me to be more directive and confrontative with him. He was motivated to learn about himself, to experience his affect, and to heal. He wanted to see results immediately. As we explored his request, we reached a compromise of sorts. I agreed to increase my degree of confrontation and employ strategies to focus him on his emotion. He recognized that he was ultimately responsible for facing his emotion and healing and that it would not occur immediately.

We also made use of our interactions in therapy to discuss how he related to people outside the therapy hour. Ryan had difficulty developing close interpersonal relationships and had been frustrated with his lack of social support. Given the models of maintaining emotional distance and control exemplified by both his father and wrestling culture, it is not surprising that Ryan protected himself in social relationships. Although it was clear that he was able to open up with me more than with others, I still experienced him as maintaining some emotional distance. He could tell me the facts, and label some feelings, but his affective expression remained flat. I used my observations and feelings as a springboard to explore how our interactions might reflect his relationships in the "real world."

One of my favorite approaches to exploring affect and one that I find most helpful is the use of immediacy in session. I employ gestalt and role playing strategies to assist clients as they experience their emotions. When Ryan began to access his emotions I encouraged him to stay with his affective states while in session rather than to avoid or resort to "brain cloud." We role played how he could respond to his former therapist, father, and mother when he confronted them. After some practice with this strategy, he would even request that I play a particular person in his life so that he could practice communicating his concerns. On other occasions, we utilized an empty chair which allowed him to "talk to" a hypothetical person in the room or the source of his anger. Sometimes I would need to confront him as he retreated into intellectualization to avoid the affect. By staying in the present, he was able to fully experience his pain on numerous occasions and to work through the pain rather than avoid it. By changing his approach to coping with pain, he began resolving some of these issues.

A little over a year into our therapy relationship, Ryan began missing appointments. He usually reported thinking that we had scheduled a different time, although once he forgot to cancel when he went out of town. I was surprised at first because Ryan had been so consistent and committed (as with his sport training). Each time he missed we would clarify the mistake and plan again. After the third time, I began to suspect that there was an issue we needed to address which was preventing him from keeping appointments. I confronted him on his recent pattern of missing sessions. We discussed his improvements in therapy, especially the reduction in his depression, and the sense that therapy was not as necessary as it had been. In addition, he was driving nearly an hour each way to my office for sessions and commented on the extra time and stress involved in such travel. I offered two possible interpretations for discussion. First, he had achieved his goals in therapy (reduction in depression) and could now consider termination. I saw a parallel between his struggle with sport retirement and therapy "retirement" and wondered if he was sending me a message about his readiness to terminate therapy. Not wanting to replay his interactions with his father regarding wrestling, I wanted to attend to this message. Second, we had done some of the relatively easy work and now were facing some more difficult issues (confronting parents) that he wished to avoid. We both agreed that there were many issues to address, and Ryan was not ready to "retire" from therapy yet. He renewed his commitment and was consistent until formal termination.

Termination of Therapy

Ryan's plans to pursue a graduate education in a different state set the stage for our termination. We both knew well in advance when he would leave, and thus we could prepare for termination. Ryan was relieved and ready to end therapy mostly because of his lengthy drive each week for the appointments. In addition, he had successfully worked through his depression and rarely reported feeling depressed, though he sometimes experienced anxiety. He was better able to express his emotions and had achieved considerable insight into the causes of his initial depression. He felt he had reached closure on the decision to retire from wrestling as well as on the breakup of his dating relationship. He had reduced his dosage of medication and was hoping eventually to stop completely. Although he noted a marked improvement, he still was fearful that he would be unable to cope with the depression if it ever reemerged.

As we discussed termination, Ryan recognized that certain issues would require further work. He had made progress in the relationships with both parents; however, he continued to struggle with defining himself in those relationships. In addition, he often held back his true feelings when in the presence of his parents and later felt "brain cloud." We also discussed body image and eating patterns as areas for further work.

During our last two sessions, we looked back at the progress in Ryan's healing and the positive nature of our therapeutic relationship. We discussed his future plans and how to cope with depression should he experience it again. I gave him the option of contacting me if any difficulties arose.

After termination, he called twice. The first time related to questioning his decision to pursue a clinical psychology graduate program and the second involved his sister's attempted suicide. We spoke briefly on the telephone each time, and after each conversation he reported having enough direction to address his concerns.

CONCLUSIONS

This case illustrates the fascinating and rewarding direction much of my sport psychology consulting has taken. I find myself more often integrating sport and personal issues than focusing purely on performance enhancement. By maintaining long-term therapeutic relationships in which the athlete can examine and express emotions, I can understand the "big picture" in an athlete's life rather than limiting myself to more circumspect performance issues. I like the complexities of understanding an athlete more completely. I also am able to observe progress over time and see that I can make a difference in the athlete's life, not just his or her sport involvement.

Often the sport issue is the initial presenting concern. As that progresses and rapport continues, the therapy evolves into examining life issues. In this case we explored family of origin issues and relationship issues that were less related to Ryan's sport involvement. In addition, we saw how the sport culture formed Ryan's identity as an athlete and person. Many of his characteristics and personal issues evolved from his training in the sport context. Ryan was able to make substantial progress in the personal realm as well as understanding the complex issues surrounding his retirement from wrestling. Work in both domains was facilitated by my combined training in the sport sciences and psychology and my credibility as a sport psychologist.

REFERENCES

Baillie, P.H.F. (1993). Understanding retirement from sports: Therapeutic ideas for helping athletes in transition. *The Counseling Psychologist, 21,* 399-410.

Blinde, E.M. & Stratta, T.M. (1992). The "sport-career death" of collegiate athletes: Involuntary and unanticipated sport exits. *Journal of Sport Behavior, 15,* 3-20.

Brownell, K.D., Steen, S.N., & Wilmore, J.H. (1987). Weight regulation practices in athletes: Analysis of metabolic and health effects. *Medicine and Science in Sports and Exercise, 19,* 546-554.

Burches-Miller, M.E. & Black, D.R. (1991). College athletes and eating disorders: A theoretical context. In D.R. Black (Ed.) *Eating disorders among athletes: Theory, Issues, and Research* (pp. 11-25). Reston, VA: American Alliance for Health, Physical Education, Recreation and Dance.

Danish, S.J., Petitpas, A.J. & Hale, B.D. (1992). A developmental-educational intervention model of sport psychology. *The Sport Psychologist, 6,* 403-415.

Danish, S.J., Petitpas, A.J. & Hale, B.D. (1993). Life development interventions for athletes: Life skills through sports. *The Counseling Psychologist, 21,* 352-385.

Greendorfer, S.L. & Blinde, E.M. (1985). "Retirement" from intercollegiate sport: Theoretical and empirical considerations. *Sociology of Sport Journal, 2,* 101-110.

Hallinan, C.J. & Snyder, E.E. (1987). Forded disengagement and the collegiate athlete. *Arena Review, 11,* 28-34.

Nitzke, S.A., Voichick, S.J., & Olson, D. (1992). Weight cycling practices and long-term health conditions in a sample of former wrestlers and other collegiate athletes. *Journal of Athletic Training, 27,* 257-261.

Ogilvie, B.C. & Howe, M. (1986). The trauma of termination from athletics. In J.M. Williams (Ed.) *Applied sport psychology: Personal growth to peak performance* (pp. 365-382). Palo Alto, CA: Mayfield Publishing Company.

Petrie, T.A., Diehl, N.S., & Watkins, C.E. Jr. (1995). Sport psychology: An emerging domain in the counseling psychology profession. *The Counseling Psychologist, 23,* 535-545.

Petrie, T.A. & Diehl, N.S. (1995). Sport psychology in the profession of psychology. *Professional Psychology: Research and Practice, 26,* 288-291.

Ravizza, K. (October, 1994). *Mental skills training for enhancing sport performance.* Association for the Advancement of Applied Sport Psychology, Lake Tahoe, Nevada.

Taylor, J.A., McCann, S.C. & Horsely, H. (October, 1994). *Identifying, describing and demonstrating practical mental skills for athletes: Sport Confidence and intensity.* Association for the Advancement of Applied Sport Psychology, Lake Tahoe, Nevada.

Taylor, J. & Schneider, B.A. (1992). The sport-clinical intake protocol: A comprehensive interviewing instrument for applied sport psychology. *Professional Psychology: Research and Practice, 23,* 318-325.

Van Raalte, J.L. & Andersen, M.B. (1996). Referral processes in sport psychology. In J.L. Van Raalte & B.W. Brewer (Eds.), *Exploring sport and exercise psychology* (pp. 275-286). Washington, DC: American Psychological Association.

A Multi-Modal Approach
to Trauma Recovery:
A Case History

N. James Bauman
Christopher M. Carr

SUMMARY. The details of a non-sport-related traumatic injury to an intercollegiate football player are presented. A multi-modal approach for treating trauma symptoms in this case history consisted of cognitive therapy, Eye Movement Desensitization and Reprocessing (EMDR), and Restricted Environmental Stimulation Technique (REST). Rationale for the treatment choices utilized is provided. A coordinated multi-modal approach effectively relieved trauma symptoms associated with this case. *[Article copies available for a fee from The Haworth Document Delivery Service: 1-800-342-9678. E-mail address: getinfo@haworth.com]*

Generally, when the topic of sport injury arises the focus of attention centers on injury sustained while participating in practice or competition (Heil, 1993; Petitpas & Danish, 1995: Weise & Troxel, 1986). Discussion then ensues regarding seriousness of the injury, possible indications for

N. James Bauman, PhD, is affiliated with the Department of Intercollegiate Athletics, Washington State University.

Christopher M. Carr, PhD, is affiliated with The Ohio State University Sports Medicine Center.

Address correspondence to: N. James Bauman, Washington State University, Department of Intercollegiate Athletics, Pullman, WA 99164-1610 (E-mail: jimb@wsu.edu).

[Haworth co-indexing entry note]: "A Multi-Modal Approach to Trauma Recovery: A Case History." Bauman, N. James, and Christopher M. Carr. Co-published simultaneously in *The Psychotherapy Patient* (The Haworth Press, Inc.) Vol. 10, No. 3/4, 1998, pp. 145-160; and: *Integrating Exercise, Sports, Movement and Mind: Therapeutic Unity* (ed: Kate F. Hays) The Haworth Press, Inc., 1998, pp. 145-160. Single or multiple copies of this article are available for a fee from The Haworth Document Delivery Service [1-800-342-9678, 9:00 a.m. - 5:00 p.m. (EST). E-mail address: getinfo@haworth.com].

medical intervention, rehabilitation regimens, and projected time to recover to full competitive levels (Arnheim, 1993; Green, 1991; Ievleva & Orlich, 1991; Petitpas & Danish, 1995; Samples, 1987). Successful recovery in the shortest time possible is central for athletes, coaches, and treatment providers. If the athlete is identified as a key player and is concurrently seen as necessary for team success, there is further pressure for a short rehabilitation period. Often, a genuine concern for the athlete's welfare can be replaced with concern over what the athlete can or can no longer provide for the good of the team.

Descriptions of injuries that involve athletes off the practice and playing fields are not found in the literature. This case history discusses a traumatic injury sustained by an intercollegiate football player in the context of his life away from sports. In the case of this athlete, full physical recovery was not possible. An interdisciplinary and multi-modal approach focused on the welfare of this athlete and the injury recovery process. Ultimately, his performance surpassed his previous athletic performances.

CASE HISTORY

The athlete involved in this case will be referred to as "PS,"[1] who is the son of first-generation immigrants from Iran. His parents settled in a large urban area where PS grew up in the innercity. His involvement in sports came late in high school. PS found that sports provided an avenue for connecting with others in the school. Sports also provided PS with a special identity often associated with those demonstrating exceptional athletic abilities. Although he had grown up in an innercity neighborhood, his involvement in sport was unlike the more stereotypical reasons for sport participation, that is, pursuing a way out of the innercity life style. Rather, PS was motivated by the work ethic passed on to him and expected by his father and grandfather. His grandfather had encouraged him to be a physician at an early age and instilled the necessary strong personal determination and hard work to realize such a pursuit. It was this same determination and work ethic that contributed to PS's successful high school football experience. However, because of his lack of size and speed relative to other major collegiate football prospects, he was not recruited by larger universities and was not offered an athletic scholarship.

PS was determined to play NCAA Division 1A football. This level of collegiate football generally includes most of the larger universities. He chose a more rural Pacific Athletic Conference (PAC-10) university to be relatively close to home, have a better probability of experiencing actual playing time, and potentially earn an athletic scholarship to defray academic expenses. He was accepted at the university and turned out for football without being recruited and without a scholarship. He demonstrated the desire and potential ability to play collegiate football and was given the opportunity to remain with the team. For three years, PS played on the junior varsity team and the "scout team." The scout team is composed of players who compete in practice against the varsity squads and play as if they are the varsity's next opponents. Often, non-scholarship athletes comprise the junior varsity and scout teams. These non-scholarship athletes invest the same amount of time and energy to the sport as scholarship athletes, without seeing much, if any, actual game experience. During PS's first and second years, he often described being ambivalent over whether or not the daily grind of time juggling the demands of pre-medicine academics and collegiate athletics was worth it. However, his motivation to continue was grounded in his basic value that hard work and determination could eventually result in achieving his goals.

Most sport fans are aware that football is a fall sport. What may not be as well known is that the spring is a significant training period for collegiate football. Spring practice, which typically lasts for five to six weeks, provides coaches with an opportunity to practice and view the team without the graduating seniors. Spring practice is just as intense and demanding of players and coaches as the fall practices. It is an opportunity for players to again try to demonstrate to coaches that they are worthy of a starting position or more playing time in the upcoming football season. It was after spring practices had concluded and in PS's third full year of being a student-athlete that this case history began to evolve into an injury-related situation.

PS had developed a friendship with another non-scholarship football player who was also pursuing an athletic scholarship. Their friendship involved motivating each other on the practice field and in the weight room, as well as socially away from athletics. PS and his friend did well in spring practice. As a result, both individuals were more likely to earn increased playing time in the fall. With spring practice concluded, the hours previously occupied by football practice opened up for other activities.

PS's friend had an interest in military special forces. The friend's interest in demolition work often associated with military special forces missions subsequently led to discussions about explosives. Their shared curiosity about the possibility of being able to make and detonate an explosive eventually led to the actual construction of an explosive device. According to PS, the plan was to simply see if they could build and detonate the mechanism. Because of the extremely rural and agricultural nature of the local geography, they intended to detonate this device in a nearby farm field. Neither individual apparently realized the magnitude of the explosive that they had constructed or the extreme danger associated with handling it.

On the way to the field, the mechanism accidentally detonated. It had been placed between PS and his friend on the front seat of the friend's vehicle. Rescue workers subsequently described the damage to the vehicle as so severe that it was miraculous that anyone had survived the blast. PS's friend was critically injured by the blast and was air-transported to a trauma unit approximately 75 miles away. PS, also seriously injured, was flown to a different trauma unit approximately 300 miles away. PS described being fully conscious during the entire ordeal. Although he admitted feeling a sense of shock and disbelief at the scene of the accident, he was fully aware of the extent of his own injuries and those to his friend. As a result of the blast, damage to PS's left hand was so extensive that amputation above the wrist was necessary. He also received extensive shrapnel and burn damage to his right hand and left leg. PS's friend's injuries were so extensive that he died after only a few days in the hospital.

THE IMMEDIATE RESPONSE

News of this kind of tragedy quickly travels through a small rural community. Further, in this farming community of approximately 25,000 people, college sports provide the majority of the local entertainment and incidents involving athletes traditionally receive wide-spread attention. Student-athletes are easily recognized by both university members and townspeople. The news that football players at a major university had been injured by an explosion became a national news story. Additionally, incidents involving explosions require federal agencies to be involved to investigate the possibility of terrorist affiliation. The news of federal involvement in this case increased the already bizarre nature of this incident in a community that is usually quiet and out of the national spotlight.

The university immediately mobilized an action plan. Most of the response resources came from university Student Affairs personnel, the Athletic Department administration, football coaches, spiritual advisors, and the sport psychologist. The parents and families of the two players were flown from their homes to the respective hospitals. Football coaches traveled in different directions to distant hospitals to be with their players and the players' families. The remaining football team members and other friends were contacted. They were given opportunities to meet with the clergy, sport psychologist, and counselors individually or in groups. Some individuals took advantage of these services, although many chose to deal with their pain in their own personal ways.

In the early stages of this tragedy, the shock and disbelief experienced by the university and the community was apparent. A few days after the university received news of PS's friend's death, a university memorial service was organized by the campus clergy. His family, the football team, other student-athletes, Athletic Department staff, and many university students and staff attended a highly emotional service. The tragedy and immediate after-effects lingered on, as evidenced by a somber university-wide graduation ceremony that took place only three weeks later.

PS's condition stabilized following a number of surgeries. He found out about his friend's death while between surgeries. Healing from injuries sustained in the blast and from the subsequent reconstructive surgery took more than three months. He was eventually fitted for a prosthesis to replace his left hand. His right hand and left leg were surgically repaired and gradually became more functional. Along with the loss of his left hand and the temporary loss of use of his right hand, PS also dealt with the loss of his good friend. He described experiencing feelings of guilt, regret, depression, confusion, anger, and hopelessness about the future. Many of these emotions were fueled by media reports and discussions by those who knew PS and his friend. Initial speculations included "why did they make the bomb," "if it was a bomb, for who or what was it intended," "how stupid they were to be messing with explosives," and "whose fault was it that the explosive detonated in the truck."

PS later talked to the first author about how emotionally overwhelmed he felt by the accident and its aftermath while in the hospital. Through all of the speculation, questions, and rehabilitation, both his family and his deceased friend's family remained in close support of him. Supporters generally attempted to be helpful by talking to PS about getting better and looking toward the future. PS described the encouragement as being difficult for him to mentally process and see as possible. He was not able to realistically see himself returning to the university at that point in his recovery. In fact, he described having a somewhat discouraged attitude about recovery and the future. He also stated that the hospital personnel attempted to provide counseling services, a response that seemed well-intended. However, rather than giving him any sense of relief, PS felt that these efforts seemed to add to his feelings of being overwhelmed. Thus, he was generally non-receptive to counseling services offered by the hospital.

RETURN TO THE UNIVERSITY

During the summer months and his initial stages of recovery, PS concluded that he must return to campus to finish what he had begun. His lengthy recovery included many hours in silent conversations with himself and with his deceased friend. Conversations were about what to do and what must be done next. Eventually, PS began to formulate commitments both for himself and to his friend's memory. These commitments included returning to the university, finishing school, regaining his physical strength, and competing in his last year of football eligibility. PS believed that if he could accomplish these things, his efforts would more accurately portray his own true character, as well as that of his deceased friend. PS was concerned that the public view of the entire incident might reinforce the sometimes stereotyped attributes associated with football players (e.g., stupid, aggressive, violent, juvenile, etc.). Instead, PS and his friend were genuinely hard workers, intelligent, risk-takers, and determined to be successful. People would never forget the tragedy, but they might remember PS's remarkable courage and hard work to re-establish a sense of respect for his deceased friend and for himself.

Along with several thousand other students, PS returned to the campus in July, the same campus that he had been air-lifted from just three months before. August represents the time of year when academic classes resume and football returns as a major source of local entertainment. Everywhere PS went on campus, he was reminded of the times before the explosion, when he and his friend would walk the campus grounds. As the first few days passed, the symptoms that PS experienced grew in number and intensity. He felt increased feelings of intense fear, recurrent and intrusive flashback episodes, and had nightmares about the incident. He described feeling constantly watched by other students. He was certain they had identified him as the football player who was involved in the explosion the previous spring. Although this may have been true, his prosthesis, as well as his large physical size compared to other students, may have made him more noticeable to others. He found himself trying to hide his prosthesis to avoid being recognized. His previous desire to be seen as a starting football player was a much different identity than the one he now possessed. He quickly realized that his plan of returning to campus and re-establishing respect was going to be much harder than he had imagined.

TREATMENT

The Athletic Department at this university created the sport psychologist position in 1986. Working full-time in the athletic department, the sport psychologist provides performance enhancement services, individual counseling, team interventions, coach consultations, crisis response, and other services typically provided by a university counseling center. Student-athletes of both genders and from all sports seek sport psychology services.

The first author's theoretical approach to counseling is primarily cognitive, based on the underlying rationale that the way individuals structure their experiences determines how they feel and behave (Beck, 1961, 1963, 1967). Cognitions are derived from beliefs, attitudes, and assumptions. The overall strategy of this therapy is a blend of verbal procedures and behavior modification techniques. These techniques are designed to help the client identify, reality test, and correct distorted conceptualizations and the dysfunctional beliefs underlying these cognitions. If the client is able to think and act more realistically and adaptively with regard to current psychological and situational problems, it is anticipated that the client will experience symptom improvement. Depending upon the presenting problems, cognitive therapy can be utilized in either a short- or long-term treatment approach.

PS had taken advantage of sport psychology services during his first year at the university. At that time, he was specifically interested in more effectively dealing with his discouragement over not playing in varsity games. This was dealt with by addressing PS's beliefs, attitudes, and assumptions about his abilities, the abilities of other players, and the probability of regularly playing in a starting role. Since PS still had three years of competitive eligibility remaining, a longer-term cognitive approach focused on motivational issues. He would also have opportunities to increase his chances of playing time by improving his physical strength, quickness, and linebacker skills.

Over the next two years (prior to the explosion), sport psychology services were utilized by the football team (e.g., setting goals, monitoring goal achievement, visualization work, etc.) and NJB would often observe practices. Contact with PS was maintained within this team setting and informally at practice. Periodically, PS would be seen for follow-up sessions just to maintain the counseling relationship and to monitor his progress.

After a few weeks back on campus following the incident and summer recovery process, PS resumed counseling with NJB. He stated that he just could not cope with all of the challenges that he was encountering with his return to campus. He also stated that he had decided to return to counseling at this time because he felt the previous assistance he received from NJB was helpful and that he definitely needed guidance again. This time, the counseling was focused on symptoms associated with what was soon diagnosed as Post-Traumatic Stress Disorder (American Psychiatric Association, 1994).

PS was obviously in a depressed state in his initial session. His symptoms included: not eating regularly, inability to concentrate in classes, decreased energy, inability to sleep, no interest in social activities, heightened feelings of irritability and anger, and an increased level of frustration over daily living tasks that he had known as a two-handed person (e.g., fastening clothing, tying shoe laces, driving a standard-shift vehicle, handling money, carrying more than one item, cooking, eating, bathing, word-processing, catching a football, etc.). He was already behind in classwork and was feeling hopeless about the future. His role with the football team was also a concern. He would not be able to participate in the fall season due to his medical condition. However, he would still be eligible to play one more year provided he were physically and psychologically ready to play the following year. Under the circumstances, rapid symptom relief was an important goal of treatment. Although cognitive therapy had previously worked well, the time involved in realizing therapeutic outcome without escalating symptoms or getting further behind in academics was a concern.

The option of psychotropic medication was presented to PS. He had strong convictions about not using medication in his current situation except as an absolute last resort. He understood the time constraints under which we were working and was open to nearly any approach that might be helpful . . . other than medication.

EYE MOVEMENT DESENSITIZATION AND REPROCESSING

A relatively new but debated procedure for treating trauma victims is known as Eye Movement Desensitization and Reprocessing (EMDR), developed by Francine Shapiro (1989a, 1989b, 1991). EMDR has been presented as an approach offering rapid and effective treatment for reducing the negative emotionality associated with traumatic memories. Initial experimental data was developed with victims of sexual assault and Vietnam veterans (Boudewyns, Stwertka, Hyer, Albrecht, & Sperr, 1993; Shapiro, 1989a, 1989b, 1991).

EMDR was becoming a more well-known form of treatment for PTSD at about the same time that PS's trauma occurred. Three licensed psychologists and a psychology doctoral intern at the university Counseling Services had all received training in EMDR and were successfully utilizing this technique. Local treatment outcome seemed to support the reported effectiveness of EMDR. After NJB consulted with these providers, EMDR procedures were introduced to PS as an alternative method for possibly reducing his symptoms in a rapid fashion. PS agreed to the procedure provided by the Counseling Center staff certified for EMDR.

The doctoral intern met with PS and NJB to explain the procedure, as well as the likelihood of positive outcome. The intern conducted seven EMDR sessions with PS. During the first two sessions, PS provided specific detail about the event and his recurring thoughts and feelings about the trauma. The remaining five sessions consisted of having PS perform rhythmic saccadic eye movements while recalling small, but sequential, pieces of the vivid details of his trauma experience. Saccadic eye movements continued until PS reported that the feelings attached to these memories had dissipated. Sessions continued until all of the negative feelings attached to the trauma event were absent. Following these five treatment sessions, nearly all of the previously reported PTSD-like and depressive symptoms were gone. The following symptom improvements were reported by PS: increased concentration, increased energy level, few to no intrusive thoughts, absence of nightmares, return of normal sleep pattern, increased appetite, increased social involvement, expanded range of affect, and excitement about the future. The effectiveness of EMDR with PS was noteworthy, as significant improvement was observed over a relatively short period of time.

CASE MANAGEMENT

The therapeutic outcome of the EMDR treatment provided PS with new perspectives and new energy to begin dealing with the challenges ahead. These included maintaining good academic standing, regaining his physical strength, becoming more adept at using his prosthesis, self-managing medical needs, establishing realistic goals for returning to football, and monitoring his psychological well-being over the coming weeks. Additional service providers were required to meet these challenges. A coordinated plan was developed that took into account the various treatment strategies, available times, and applicable timeframes of all individuals involved. After some discussion, PS and NJB decided that it would be therapeutic for him to be more active in managing his treatment needs. NJB assisted with contacting appropriate resources and monitoring the progression of the recovery process. An important reason to place PS in a position of increased control was to establish a mindset that he was a capable person, rather than one who was disabled. He responded well to this challenge.

Resources were identified and PS initiated the contacts. For example, he contacted adaptive physical education instructors to design specific strength programs for his left arm to minimize muscle atrophy in his forearm. These programs primarily consisted of swimming pool workouts with paddles strapped to his arm. He contacted the Director of Athletic Medicine and established a relationship with a single trainer to work with his rehabilitation. Working with an amputee-athlete was a new experience for athletic medicine staff. PS also contacted the School of Mechanical and Materials Engineering on campus and the Assistant Strength and Conditioning Coach to cooperatively develop a prototype prosthesis attachment to replace the standardized "pincher" attachment. The new attachment was necessary to accommodate lifting weights. He was introduced to a graduate student in mechanical engineering who developed a master's thesis project out of constructing the new prosthetic attachment.

RESTRICTED ENVIRONMENTAL STIMULATION TECHNIQUE (REST)

PS made significant progress in both his physical and psychological conditions over a five-month period. His goals of finishing school, possibly competing in his last year of football eligibility, and re-establishing an identity more associated with dedicated work ethic, rather than that of a trauma survivor, began to seem realistically attainable. In order for him to have an opportunity to play football in the fall season, he would have to demonstrate an ability to participate in the upcoming spring practice, like any other player. At this point in his recovery, spring practice was only two months away.

To evaluate a variety of strength and skill levels associated with football, spring practice includes several agility and strength tests that each athlete must complete to evaluate a variety of strength and skill levels associated with football. These tests include vertical jump, 10/20/30/40 yard sprints, bench press, and squat. Coaches established height, time, and weight standards for these tests consistent with skills associated with various positions in football. PS was making good progress, but was still some distance away from meeting the minimum test standards expected by the coaches.

As time began to run out in terms of being prepared for spring practice and being tested, PS started to feel somewhat distressed over the likelihood of meeting the minimum test expectations. As a result, he also started to lose his training focus and his progress began to plateau. It was at this time that PS was introduced to another treatment approach known as

Restricted Environmental Stimulation Technique (REST). NJB had previous research experience with REST in a sport context (Barabasz, Barabasz, & Bauman, 1993) and was concurrently working on a second REST study.

REST's antecedents are found in the early research on sensory deprivation or sensory isolation (Krivitsky, 1939; Lifton, 1961; Lilly, 1956; Zubek, 1969). The use of REST in sport began to emerge in a project conducted by Stanley and Mahoney (1987) working with improving the performance of football players. Since that original project, only six subsequent studies had been conducted utilizing flotation REST as a performance enhancing technique, in spite of its demonstrated ability to outperform other more commonly used mental skill training procedures (Barabasz, Barabasz, & Bauman, 1993; Bauman, Barabasz, & Barabasz, 1995; Lee & Hewitt, 1987; McAleney, Barabasz, & Barabasz, 1990; Suedfeld & Bruno, 1990; Wagaman, Barabasz, & Barabasz, 1991).

Freedom from external distracters has been shown to enhance one's ability to focus attention on task-relevant internally generated activity (e.g., a perfect gymnastic routine, highjumping, skiing, marksmanship, etc.). REST provides a comfortable environment that restricts external sensory stimulation.

The technique utilized with PS is more specifically known as dry flotation REST. In dry flotation REST, subjects lie supine on a pliable polymer membrane contained within a rectangular wooden chamber. The wooden chamber is sound attenuated, eliminates light, and provides a ventilated environment. More detailed information about dry flotation REST chamber and protocol can be found in Barabasz, Barabasz, and Bauman (1993).

Three 50-minute dry flotation sessions (one per week) were conducted with PS. The number and spacing of flotation sessions was determined in part by previous reported research and in part by time strictures. No guided imagery was conducted during the session. McAleney et al. (1990) had found that the verbal stimulus of providing imagery messages during the REST session was distracting to athletes. Prior to the first REST session, PS was simply told to imagine himself benchpressing the desired amount of weight. The next day, PS reported that he had set a personal best for the benchpress. The second and third REST sessions were geared more for the spring practice final game. Prior to these sessions, PS was told to imagine himself being quick and reactive in agility or actual football situations. PS reported having gotten feedback from his coaches that this spring practice was his best.

PS continued to participate in strength and conditioning programs. As his strength continued to improve, the prosthetic attachment for lifting weights had to be redesigned to withstand the increased weight that he was lifting.

MEDICAL CONSIDERATIONS

PS's medical progress was monitored by a Certified Athletic Trainer within the athletic department under the supervision of the neuro-surgeon who had performed the original surgeries. No medical complications developed as a result of surgery or during the course of rehabilitation. However, PS's return to football required developing special padding to protect his sensitive stump from pain associated with full contact. PS played the linebacker position where contact happened on every play. The prosthetics physician, who originally had fitted PS with a prosthesis, designed and fitted PS's left arm with protective padding to reduce the pain associated with the physical contact of football. The Director of Athletic Medicine ensured that PS's padding was fitted properly prior to practices and competitions.

PS's SENIOR YEAR

PS and NJB continued to meet approximately one to two times per month over his final year at the university. Sessions generally focused on his continuing physical and emotional progress. At times, PS would express disappointment over not getting the amount of playing time that he felt he deserved—a not-uncommon perspective of athletes, regardless of their situation. In spite of this disappointment, PS regularly talked about his progress and personal satisfaction with his overall recovery and accomplishments. During this last year, PS reported continued absence of the trauma symptoms that he previously experienced.

PS completed his last year at the university with a sense of resolve and success in several ways. The legal aspect of this case was closed by the federal agency investigating the incident. Investigators found no evidence that the explosive had been constructed for any purpose other than curiosity or excitement. PS had physically recovered from the accident. He successfully completed the requirements of the academic courses that he had been unable to finish the previous spring, due to hospitalization. In addition to making up previous course requirements, he also successfully passed full academic loads for both of his senior year semesters. Despite his prosthetic attachment, he surpassed his previous strength standards in football. He was actively involved in football practices, competed in the last game of the season, and played in a post-season bowl game. As a tribute and as a memorial to his deceased friend, PS put his friend's initials on the back of his helmet and he wore his friend's jersey number in practice and on game days. He had gained the respect of other athletes, coaches, administrators, professors, and sport fans for his determination to face academic, athletic, physical, emotional, and social challenges.

At the end-of-the-year football awards ceremony, PS was awarded the team inspirational award, the school strength award, and a special award given to those athletes who have shown exceptional courage in adverse situations. PS graduated from the university and is currently coaching collegiate linebackers. He is taking graduate courses and plans on pursuing a career as a healthcare professional. He also plans to continue working with athletes, as well as marketing new prosthetic attachments for amputee weight lifting.

REFLECTIONS

This case history describes a student-athlete who experienced a non-sport-related injury. Although his physical and emotional challenges were briefly described, the intensity of this experience is known only to PS. The challenges that faced NJB and other healthcare providers were also unique. None of the athletic department staff (e.g., coaches, athletic medicine, or strength and conditioning coaches) had previous experience with amputees. Therefore, what to do and how to coordinate treatment strategies were new experiences that we shared with PS.

The response to a tragedy of this magnitude affects the people within an athletic department to a greater degree and in a different way than the community at large. Compared to the community, the athletic department staff relationships with athletes are characterized by contacts that are more frequent, are often personal in nature, and are primarily associated with more contexts than just game day. Generally, the relationship between staff and athletes is inspired more by a common purpose and less by the awe of athleticism. Therefore, when a tragedy involves one of our athletes, it seems to feel more like one of us who has been hurt, rather than someone we know from a distance on the competitive field or through the media.

The first major obstacle to contend with in this case was that of being able to identify and process how this type of tragedy affected other athletes and athletic department staff. This included: reactions to learning of the crisis; becoming aware of the details of how this crisis occurred; going through a period of time where the conditions of both athletes were unknown; dealing with the subsequent death of one of the athletes; waiting to know whether or not PS would return to campus; if he did return, identifying his needs and formulating effective treatment plans for challenges with which we had no previous experience; and following through with services until a planned termination had been realized.

After PS made the decision to return to campus, the second major task was to begin an extensive search for local resources. Initially, contacts and consultations were made with the University Counseling Center, Department of Physical Education, local physicians, and local private practitioners. Eventually, PS's medical needs were coordinated by the Director of Athletic Medicine. His physical conditioning and rehabilitation were jointly implemented and monitored by Athletic Medicine and the Athletic Department strength and conditioning coach. Individuals from the Adaptive Physical Education Program assisted in the initial rehabilitation efforts. The development of prosthesis attachments was coordinated with the Department of Mechanical Engineering and the Athletic Department strength and conditioning coach. Counseling services were provided by NJB with frequent consults with the sport psychologist (CC) and other psychologists from the University Counseling Center. Although a number of scheduling conflicts were encountered with so many service providers, everyone maintained an exceptional level of flexibility so that services could be developed, coordinated, delivered, and monitored. Significant factors contributing to the cooperation of those involved may have included the nature of the trauma, a "small-town" atmosphere, the qualities of the providers, and PS's active participation in his own case management.

It has now been more than four years since the accident and two years since PS graduated from the university. NJB and PS continue to have periodic telephone contacts. The anniversary date of the accident provides an annual reminder to PS. Telephone contact is made with PS on or about the anniversary date for continued support and to inquire about his continuing progress. PS's case illustrates the benefits of putting an athlete's welfare first and not being hesitant to try innovative approaches to new challenges. It illustrates how a coordinated, multi-disciplined, and multimodal approach can be helpful to athletes.

NOTE

1. The client-athlete involved in this case history has provided his input, as well as his authorization to share his experience in hopes of assisting other athletes in their recovery process and to encourage healthcare providers to be creative helpers.

REFERENCES

American Psychiatric Association: *Diagnostic and Statistical Manual of Mental Disorders, Fourth Edition*. Washington, DC, American Psychiatric Association, 1994.

Arnheim, D. (1993). *Principles of athletic training, 8th edition*. St. Louis.

Barabasz, A. (1990). Restricted environmental stimulation enhances concentration and performance in formula car race driving: A case study. Attentional Processes Laboratory Reports, Washington State University, October.

Barabasz, A., Barabasz, M., & Bauman, J. (1993). Restricted environmental stimulation technique improves human performance: Rifle marksmanship. *Perceptual and Motor Skills, 76*, 867-873.

Bauman, J., Barabasz, A., & Barabasz, M. (1995). Effects of dry and wet flotation restricted environmental stimulation interventions on attentional processes and performance. Unpublished dissertation. Washington State University.

Beck, A. T. (1961). A systematic investigation of depression. *Comprehensive Psychiatry, 2*, 162-170.

Beck, A. T. (1963). Thinking and depression. *Archives of General Psychiatry, 9*, 324-333.

Beck, A. T. (1967). *Depression*. New York: Hoeber-Harper.

Boudewyns, P. S., Stwertka, S. A., Hyer, L. A., Albrecht, J. W., & Sperr, E. V., (1993). Eye movement desensitization for PTSD of combat: A treatment outcome pilot study. *The Behavior Therapist, 16*, 29-33.

Green, L. (1992). The use of imagery in the rehabilitation of athletes. *The Sports Psychologist*, 416-428.

Heil, J. (1993). *Psychology of sport injury*. Champaign, IL.

Hutchinson, B. (1984). *The book of floating*. New York: Ronald.

Ievleva, L. & Orlich, T. (1991). Mental links to enhanced healing: An exploratory study. *The Sports Psychologist, 5*, (1), 25-40.

Krivitsky, W. (1939). *In Stalin's secret service*. New York: Harper.

Lee, A. & Hewitt, J. (1987). Using visual imagery in a flotation tank to improve gymnastic performance and reduce physical symptoms. *International Journal of Sports Psychology, 18*, 223-230.

Lifton, R. (1961). *Thought reform and the psychology of totalism*. NY: Norton.

Lilly, J. C. (1956). Mental effects of reduction of ordinary levels of physical stimuli on intact, healthy persons. *Psychiatric Research Reports, 5*, 1-9.

McAleney, P., Barabasz, A., & Barabasz, M. (1990). The effects of flotation restricted environmental stimulation on intercollegiate tennis performance. *Perceptual and Motor Skills, 71*, 1023-1028.

Morgan, A. & Kilgard, J. R. (1975). Stanford hypnotic clinical scale. In E. R. Hilgard & J. R. Hilgard (Eds.), *Hypnosis in the relief of pain* (pp. 209-221). Los Altos, CA: Kaufman.

Petitpas, A. & Danish, S. J. (1995). Caring of injured athletes. In Murphy, S. M. (Ed.). *Sport psychology interventions* (255-278). Human Kinetics.

Samples, P. (1987). Mind over muscles: Returning the injured athlete to play. *Physical Sports Medicine, 15*, (10), 172-180.

Shapiro, F. (1989a). Efficacy of the eye movement desensitization procedure in the treatment of traumatic memories. *Journal of Traumatic Stress, 2,* 199-223.

Shapiro, F. (1989b). Eye movement desensitization: A new treatment for post-traumatic stress disorder. *Journal of Behavior Therapy and Experimental Psychiatry, 20,* 211-217.

Shapiro, F. (1991). Eye movement desensitization and reprocessing procedure: From EMD to EMD/R–A new model for anxiety and related trauma. *The Behavior Therapist, 13,* 133-135.

Stanley, J., Mahoney, M. & Reppert, S. (1987). REST and the enhancement of sports performance: A panel presentation and discussion. In J. W. Turner, Jr. & T. H. Fine (Eds.). *Proceedings of the 2nd International Conference on REST* (pp. 168-183). Toledo, OH; International REST Investigator's Society.

Suedfeld, P. & Bruno, T. (1990). Flotation REST and imagery in the improvement of athletic performance. *Journal of Sport and Exercise Psychology, 12,* 82-85.

Suedfeld, P., Collier, D. & Hartnett, B. (1993). Enhancing perceptual motor accuracy through flotation REST. *Sport Psychologist, 7,* 151-159.

Wagaman, J., Barabasz, A., & Barabasz, M. (1991). Flotation REST and imagery in the improvement of collegiate basketball performance. *Perceptual and Motor Skills, 72,* 119-122.

Weise, M. R. & Troxel, R. K. (1986). Psychology of the injured athlete. *Athletic Training, 21,* 104-109.

Anxiety Management
and the Elite Athlete:
A Case Study

Trent A. Petrie

SUMMARY. In this paper, therapeutic work with an elite, African-American female athlete is described. The focus of treatment was threefold: (1) anxiety management; (2) relationships with coach; and (3) race and social isolation. Strategies used to address each issue are described, as is the general outcome for this athlete. *[Article copies available for a fee from The Haworth Document Delivery Service: 1-800-342-9678. E-mail address: getinfo@haworth.com]*

Mary T. is a 30-year-old, African-American woman who was a competitive volleyball and softball player in high school. Although she did not pursue these sports in college, she remained physically active. Following completion of her undergraduate education, she became interested in her current sport, cycling, and began to train and compete on her own. Due to her athletic talent and hard work, over the next few years Mary was successful in local and regional amateur competitions. As a result of these successes, a professional coach offered to train her as part of his team. During the first year of professional coaching, which included all aspects of her training (e.g., weight lifting, nutrition, biomechanics), Mary's strength, physical stamina, and performances improved significantly. In

Trent A. Petrie, PhD, is affiliated with the Department of Psychology, P.O. Box 13587, University of North Texas, Denton, TX 76203 (E-mail: TPETRIE@ VM.ACS.UNT.EDU).

[Haworth co-indexing entry note]: "Anxiety Management and the Elite Athlete: A Case Study." Petrie, Trent A. Co-published simultaneously in *The Psychotherapy Patient* (The Haworth Press, Inc.) Vol. 10, No. 3/4, 1998, pp. 161-173; and: *Integrating Exercise, Sports, Movement and Mind: Therapeutic Unity* (ed: Kate F. Hays) The Haworth Press, Inc., 1998, pp. 161-173. Single or multiple copies of this article are available for a fee from The Haworth Document Delivery Service [1-800-342-9678, 9:00 a.m. - 5:00 p.m. (EST). E-mail address: getinfo@haworth.com].

fact, her coach was so pleased with her progress that his goal for her became national and international competitions.

Unfortunately, the next two years were disappointing: Mary failed to achieve the performances and successes that had been anticipated. She had performance successes (e.g., personal bests) in road races. In sprint competitions, however, she experienced noticeable decrements due primarily to two factors: (a) overwhelming anxiety prior to and at the beginning of competition and (b) the lack of a "killer" instinct during competition, which she attributed to precompetitive anxiety. She ended the season very frustrated with her inability to win major competitions or place consistently at the top. Her coach began to question her abilities and his plans for her. In addition to this external stress, Mary experienced internal pressure to be successful because she was one of only a few African-American women competing at this level in her sport. Upon determining that she could not handle another year of disappointments and that she was not improving on her own, Mary contacted me during the fall for assistance.

THE INITIAL INTAKE AND EVALUATION PROCESS

Mary entered the first session reporting a wide assortment of physical and psychological symptoms of anxiety, including muscle tension, racing heart, upset stomach, and poor concentration, that had progressively worsened during the last two competitive seasons. Her initial reports suggested that her primary problems were anxiety and performing poorly, generally considered performance enhancement issues. However, it also was important and necessary to thoroughly explore nonsport related areas to ascertain her overall level of social/personal functioning and determine the best way to intervene. Using the Sport-Clinical Intake Protocol (Taylor & Schneider, 1992) as a guide, we discussed the following areas in depth: presenting problem, sport performance history, family and social support, general health, important life events in the recent past, changes temporally related to the presenting problem, and race/ethnicity.

As noted above, Mary's presenting problem was the experience of extremely high levels of anxiety that interfered significantly with her ability to compete. Further exploration revealed that she was in top physical condition, and under the care of her team's exercise and nutritional specialists. We discussed the issue of staleness (Morgan, Brown, Raglin, O'Connor, & Ellickson, 1987) to determine if any of her psychological symptoms were related to overtraining. She reported being aware of the phenomenon and, given that this was the off-season with a relatively light training load, did not believe that it might be contributing to her current situation or symptoms. Although her job and training regimen allowed little time for socializing, she described her personal relationships as quite satisfactory though limited to a few close friends. Her family, who she described as very close and caring, was her primary support system. She was in frequent contact over the phone and visited them as often as possible. She described her job environment as exciting and challenging.

Her teammates also were supportive, though they generally did not socialize with one another outside of the time spent together training and competing. She described her coach as fair but demanding, a man who had motivated and helped her become an accomplished performer. An aspect of the coach-athlete relationship that she found disappointing, and at times problematic, was the manner in which he gave feedback about performances. In fact, Mary was still bothered by some comments the coach had made to her following disappointing competitions the previous season. She indicated that she would like to discuss their relationship and develop the skills to communicate with him more openly and not to be as emotionally affected by his comments.

As trust and rapport were established, details surrounding the evolution of Mary's anxiety gradually emerged. From her standpoint, the anxiety had developed slowly over the course of the last two seasons (about one and a half years) though its inception could be linked to a series of particularly bad performances the previous spring. At subsequent competitions she became more aware of her physical sensations (e.g., muscle tightness, breathing), and began to interpret them in a more negative fashion (e.g., "my muscles feel really tight, I must not be ready to compete"). This cycle of negative appraisals of situations and physical sensations was reinforced by continuing poor performances, particularly in the sprint events in which the anxiety symptoms had first emerged. Over the next year, her anxiety expanded to the point that she would begin to feel nauseous two days before the competition.

Although it is not essential for the therapist to have a personal background in sport, it is necessary to have some knowledge and awareness of the dynamics of athletes and athletic competition (Cogan & Petrie, 1996). As an ex-collegiate athlete and coach and as a sport psychology professional, I had extensive knowledge of sport, athletics, and the psychological aspects of performance. I was only minimally knowledgeable, however, of the specifics of competitive cycling. Thus, I needed to educate myself about the details and dynamics of being a cyclist (e.g., training, competitions). Some of the information I obtained on my own through reading (e.g., books, sport magazines). The remainder came from Mary, who was very open and willing to provide me with details. This process served several purposes in our work. First, it demonstrated my openness and willingness to learn from her, who I viewed as the expert on herself and her sport. Second, it helped to further develop the trust and rapport of our relationship. Third, it helped me to become aware of the specific details I needed to accurately understand her experience. I now could "talk the talk." Finally, it provided us with a starting point and some direction in terms of what she wanted to attain in her psychological preparation.

Some of the information was provided in session as we discussed her anxiety and performances (e.g., she would answer technical questions about the sport). The remainder was gleaned from videotapes of her own performances as well as other cyclists who she wanted to emulate. I have found that behavioral observation of the athlete and their performances is an integral part of diagnosis and treatment planning. Through such observation, important information can be gained that athletes are unable, or perhaps unwilling, to self-report (e.g., with whom do they interact prior to competition, is this related to their performances). In addition, details about the competitive environment that may influence the manner in which a treatment is implemented can be determined (e.g., what opportunities are available before the beginning of competition for implementation of anxiety management strategies). Although I would have preferred to watch Mary compete live, because she was in the off-season we were unable to do that. The videotape provided the next best alternative.

Finally, race/ethnicity was discussed. Mary raised this issue when describing the pressures she felt. As one of only a few African-American women in her sport, Mary felt a responsibility to the sport as well as to the African-American community to be a role model and to perform at her best. Even so, she wondered if some of the expectations her coach and the sport governing body officials had of her were influenced by her race (i.e., it was important for the sport to have an African-American woman doing well). Mary herself appeared very grounded and secure in her racial identity, in the stage Helms (1983) defined as "internalization." As such, she was aware of the possibility that racial bias might exist and open to discussing the issue. She appeared to appreciate my broaching the topic and my willingness to discuss it further as our work progressed.

Given these racially related concerns, it was likewise important for us to discuss our own racial and gender differences and what effects, if any, those would have on our working together. Mary expressed comfort with our relationship and appreciated my willingness to discuss these issues. I, too, was comfortable working with Mary and aware that race was intricately woven into our social fabric and played a part in most interactions.

We did not directly address our race and gender at any later point in therapy, yet the initial openness we established allowed us to effectively discuss the above mentioned issues during later sessions.

In those instances where an athlete may have difficulty communicating the details of his/her situation, paper and pencil assessments may be useful. However, any information obtained from such assessments should be directly relevant to the athlete and be communicated in an understandable manner. It is important for consultants to have a rationale for the assessment procedures they select and to allow this selection to be guided by the specific environment and athletes with whom they are working (Cogan & Petrie, 1996). I chose to gather information from Mary primarily through interview and discussion, rather than relying on standardized assessments, as she was quite insightful and articulate about the problems she was experiencing.

As mentioned previously, I view athlete-clients as the experts on themselves and as partners in the therapy process (Cogan & Petrie, 1996). I openly share my perceptions about their concerns, involve them in the treatment planning, and answer questions they may have about me as a psychologist working with athletes or about their case in particular. This approach seems to be particularly important with athletes who already may feel stigmatized because they are seeing a psychologist (Linder, Pillow, & Reno, 1989). By openly discussing the problems and involving them in treatment, therapy becomes less mysterious and secretive and more inviting. Recent research provides initial support for this approach, finding that athletes appear to value a directive and concrete approach from therapists who are willing to openly discuss the athletes' cases and share information about themselves and their work (Miller & Moore, 1993).

GOAL SETTING AND INTERVENTION

As Mary and I defined several specific treatment goals, I identified appropriate interventions for each concern. The primary goal was learning to manage the debilitating anxiety she was experiencing in relation to her sport performance. The past poor performances were weighing heavily on Mary and she was highly motivated to work on this problem. The second major goal concerned her relationship with her coach. She wanted to be able to talk more openly with him about their relationship and her training, as well as express how his feedback affected her and her subsequent performances. The final goal concerned the issue of race and its relationship to her involvement in her sport.

When considering intervention options, two issues, timing and motivation, are especially germane. First, at what point in the athlete's competitive schedule is he/she coming to see you? Are there environmental pressures for the athlete to "get better" and start performing well immediately? In this case, Mary had just ended her competitive season and would not begin competing again until the following spring. This provided us with a window of six months during which we could work on her psychological skills training concurrently with her physical conditioning and sport training. Thus, any changes we made in how she prepared psychologically for competition could be practiced and incorporated into her physical training without the immediate pressure to compete in an important meet. Although athletes do not always seek assistance at such opportune times as did Mary, it is important to be sensitive to timing issues and how one's interventions fall in relation to upcoming competitions.

Second, what is the athlete's level of motivation for mental training? Some athletes may want a "quick fix" and not realize that, like physical training, some improvements may take time to be realized. Being clear with athletes about expected time expenditures, realistic outcomes, and potential roadblocks is crucial. Mary entered therapy highly motivated and maintained this drive throughout our work together. She understood that she was not going to reach the level of performance she desired without changing her behavioral and psychological reactions to competition. Even though she expressed high levels of interest and drive at the beginning, I was explicit that she would need to spend time outside of session to realize the changes she wanted.

Finally, whether an athlete's issue appears to be more "clinical" or "performance related," I work with them in my role as a psychologist. Thus, confidentiality is an issue that needs to be discussed. Many athletes (and nonathletes for that matter) may be unfamiliar with the concept and limits of confidentiality in a professional relationship and how these can be influenced by "who is the client." It is important that confidentiality be explained to the athlete in detail and expectations that athletes or coaches might have about communicating information concerning the psychological treatment be discussed. Because Mary was self-referred and paying on her own, I considered her the client. We discussed disclosures that would be necessary in order for her to file her insurance, general limits of confidentiality, and what would need to happen (i.e., signing release forms) should she want me to talk with her coach.

Goal I: Anxiety Management

In deciding how to treat Mary's anxiety, I considered two important factors. First, the anxiety was intense, had developed over a two year period, and involved both somatic and cognitive components. Second, she needed an anxiety management skill that was transportable, under her control, and effective not only in reducing physical components of anxiety but also in helping her refocus her thoughts. Given these considerations, I chose to teach her cue-controlled relaxation (CCR; Russell, Miller, & June, 1975) to be used in concert with systematic desensitization. CCR would provide Mary with a technique for rapid, unobtrusive, *in vivo* reduction of excessive muscle tension and interruption of negative self-defeating thoughts. She could then re-focus on more positive self-enhancing ones that would help improve performance.

CCR initially involves learning progressive muscle relaxation (PMR; Bernstein & Borkevec, 1973). Because PMR can be difficult to practice without external guidance, I encouraged Mary to tape our sessions and then use the tape to lead her through the relaxation routine at home. During the first three weeks Mary was taken through progressive muscle relaxation training during our weekly sessions with instructions to practice at home once a day during the remainder of the week. With this schedule of at-home practice, she would become proficient at relaxing herself and would experience a deeper state of relaxation. During the fourth week of PMR, the cue-word strategy was introduced. Cue-words that are one syllable, relaxation focused (e.g., "calm"), and personally meaningful, tend to be most effective. Immediately following PMR and while deeply relaxed, for about two minutes, Mary would subvocalize the cue word she chose ("win") in synchrony with each exhalation. This process was repeated after a one-minute break during which Mary visualized a relaxing scene. Mary continued to practice PMR and cue-word association, both in session and alone (following the at-home schedule described above), for the next four weeks. Based on the principles of classical conditioning, the process of pairing the cue-word with a deeply relaxed state provided Mary with the means for inducing relaxation by simply repeating her cue-word to herself.

In addition to the above training, we incorporated performance-related visualizations and identified positive, performance-enhancing thinking that could substitute for the negative thoughts associated with her anxiety. During the first four weeks of the relaxation training, Mary visualized neutral (i.e., nonsport related), soothing scenes to facilitate relaxation and assist her in becoming competent with this imagery. Over the next four weeks we extended the visualizations to neutral performance related scenes (e.g., practicing her sport). Thus, Mary became proficient with visualization of both performance and nonperformance related scenes.

About this time we also began to develop the anxiety hierarchy related to the event in which she was experiencing debilitating anxiety. The final hierarchy consisted of 15 anxiety-provoking situations related to the sprint competitions, ranging from low to high anxiety, grouped into four sets. The first set consisted of three situations that generally occurred two days before the race when she would first arrive in the city where the competition was to be held. The next set was comprised of practice situations she and her teammates would have the day before the race. The third set concerned preparation for competition the day of the meet, while the fourth set involved situations ranging from an hour before the race until it started.

At the end of the eighth week, following completion of CCR, we began the actual desensitization procedure. At this point in our work together, Mary reported feeling more relaxed and less bothered by negative, unfocused thinking during her training. Even so, Mary still recognized the need to more directly address the anxiety associated with the specific event, sprint races. Over the course of the next five sessions, we worked through the hierarchy addressing one set per session (with the exception of the last set on which we spent two sessions). As before, Mary audiotaped the sessions so she could practice effectively at home. Mary experienced no anxiety while visualizing any part of the hierarchy and, by the end, reported feeling very relaxed and confident about her performances.

In addition to the desensitization, we developed a precompetitive routine for performances that incorporated the use of her cue-word ("win"). She identified the times during which she would need to reduce her anxiety level and become focused on and confident about her performance. Because she wanted to feel powerful, in control, quick, and focused, we incorporated these words into the visualizations so she could recreate the state she wanted in actual competition. As the desensitization progressed, I encouraged her to begin using her precompetitive routine in her practices to determine its in vivo effectiveness.

As a result of the time and energy she devoted to practicing these behavioral techniques outside of session, Mary (a) became more relaxed overall, (b) developed a specific skill to reduce her muscle tension and to refocus her thinking, one that she could implement whenever she wanted (e.g., sport or nonsport situations), (c) developed a specific precompetition performance routine, and (d) increased her level of self-confidence about her sport abilities and performances by focusing on more positive, performance enhancing words and phrases as opposed to the negative ones that previously interfered. Overall, Mary indicated having great success with her routine and felt extremely confident about her abilities. In addition, she reported significant improvements in all aspects of her training; coaches and teammates noticed and commented upon these changes as well.

I find it is very useful to maintain contact with the athlete as they transfer what they have learned and practiced during the training season into competition. Sometimes the pressure of competition is more than what was experienced in practice and some additional work needs to be done to make sure the skills generalize or transfer. Ideally, Mary and I would have continued to work together through the beginning of the next competitive season. Unfortunately, Mary experienced a physical injury about one month before the beginning of the competitive season and needed to spend her time on physical rehabilitation and preparation. She expressed confidence in herself and what she had learned, and said that she would continue to practice relaxation and visualization one day a week to remain focused and sharp. With her injury, visualization took on a new function. It became a part of her training now that she was physically restricted. I too was confident in her progress and we ended our work together with the understanding that she could return in the succeeding months should she need any assistance.

Goal II: Relationship with Coach

The coach often occupies a central position in an athlete's life. In this instance, Mary's coach had dedicated considerable time and energy to her training over the years and had given her the opportunity to compete at her current elite level. She wanted to have a mutual level of respect and understanding, and be able to communicate her thoughts and feelings as they related to her training and their relationship. When Mary began working with me, she was distressed by the manner in which the coach tended to give her feedback about her performances. Although she understood that he was not trying to be negative, the words he used sometimes hurt her emotionally and seemed to question her motivation and desire.

By the fourth session, we were devoting less time to relaxation training and thus were able to cover other salient issues. Thus, we began to discuss the relationship with her coach. First, we identified the key event from last season that was still distressing (i.e., comments made after a poor sprint race). Second, we determined how she wanted to define the relationship now. Third, we discussed her options for coping with this situation (e.g., avoid it, talk with coach). Mary decided to set up an individual meeting with him to talk about last season as well as other issues. Prior to the meeting with her coach, we role played the interchange to provide Mary an opportunity to practice saying what she wanted. Mary found the role play helpful in that it performed a desensitizing function, allowing her to feel less anxious and more confident in her ability to discuss the issues with him.

Their meeting was successful. The coach had been unaware of the impact he had on Mary and expressed appreciation for the feedback. They were able to discuss the mutual frustrations they were feeling about her performances during the last two years. In addition, Mary shared with him that she was working with me to address her performance anxieties. As a result of this discussion, they were able to reestablish a closer, more open, and more respectful working relationship. In addition, they again focused on Mary's training and performance goals for the upcoming competitive season. She mentioned the possibility of the coach joining her in one of our sessions, yet the need never arose. Mary felt confident in their interactions and respected by him.

Goal III: Social Isolation

As one of the few African-American women in her sport, Mary felt an added responsibility to succeed and be a good role model for the African-American community. She also wondered if the attention she received in her sport was because of her race, and felt isolated in not having other African-American women with whom she could talk about such pressures. In our first meeting I broached the subject of race and how it might play a role in her sport. This was an important opening for later discussions we would have about the issue.

First, in a sport dominated by Caucasian athletes, Mary was aware that having a visibly successful minority athlete would be important for the sport from a public relations standpoint. Thus, she wondered if the high expectations her coach and officials in the sport's governing body had for her were influenced by her race. Second, because there were few other minority women in her sport, talking about these and other issues with athletes who might not be sensitive to the implications of race or have had similar experiences to her was difficult. As a result, she felt isolated. Finally, our gender and racial differences paralleled those with her coach and I wanted to be sure she was comfortable working with me.

Although there were few identifiable African-American women within her sport with whom she could develop a supportive relationship, we discussed women in other sports who were in parallel situations. In doing so, Mary expanded the possibilities of her social network and realized that there were other women with similar experiences from whom she could receive support if she desired. She also recognized that the racial aspects of the expectations were very subtle and were not in actuality interfering with her training or performances. Characteristically, she decided to not spend any time or energy on the issue, and noted that, given her improved relationship with her coach, she would be willing and able to pursue such issues should they become problematic for her.

FOLLOW-UP

As mentioned previously, Mary sustained a physical injury that required her to suspend psychological treatment. At that time we had completed our work on her three goals and were moving to monthly sessions to monitor her progress as she entered the competitive season. Mary expressed a high level of satisfaction with her treatment and believed that she was performing better in training than she had in previous years. She also reported feeling in control with respect to managing her anxiety prior to and during performances. Even so, it was important to maintain contact with Mary when she entered the competitive season. The work we had done appeared to be successful, yet she had not used these skills in live, competitive situations. Thus, the actual generalizability of the skills and appropriateness of the precompetitive routine remained in need of in vivo testing.

During the first month of the competitive season we were in contact through one telephone call during which Mary reported successes in her performances and generalization of the skills. She indicated that she was comfortable with her precompetitive routine and had experienced no anxiety during the event in question. At the beginning of the third month of competition, Mary experienced another injury that required her to miss subsequent meets. Toward the end of her physical rehabilitation for this recent injury, Mary contacted me for an appointment before she traveled to the national championships.

As the season progressed, Mary had noticed a problem in her performances—she was too relaxed during sprint races. As she explained it, she did not have the "killer instinct" that she desired. This problem had existed prior to beginning our work together, yet it had been overshadowed by the extreme anxiety she was experiencing. Not having the "killer instinct" was now more salient given that she no longer experienced distress due to precompetitive anxiety.

During the session, we focused on how she wanted to feel, both psychologically and physically, while competing. We identified situations in the race that she could use as environmental cues and associated meaningful words with them (i.e., ready, attack, punch it). These words represented the psychological and physical states she wanted to attain. Using visualization, we then practiced using these words in conjunction with the environmental cues during competition. Although identification and use of the words had been successful in-session, we were not sure if that would transfer to actual competition. We discussed how she could use this strategy during her training/practice sessions to facilitate generalization. I also made myself available to Mary by phone, should she have any questions concerning her performances while at the training center and then at the national championships.

I did not hear from Mary again until about three months later. During a phone conversation, Mary reported being very pleased with the work she had accomplished with me and with her performances during the year. Although she did not make the finals in her event, she set a personal record at the national championships. She reported feeling no anxiety prior to or during competition and was able to generalize to competition the "psyching up" strategy we developed in session. As I do with all my clients, we ended our work together with the opportunity for Mary to return should she need any additional assistance in the future.

CONCLUSION

This case illustrates the interaction of three important factors: expectations, goals, and personality. Initially, it is important to clarify the athletes' expectations for treatment and outcome and to realistically present time commitments and potential benefits from the outset. In addition, it is useful to clearly define the goals for working together and to directly link the work done in session to the attainment of those goals. As most athletes are familiar with and use goal setting in physical training, such an approach is likely to be consistent with their previous experience. Even with clearly established expectations and goals, the athlete's personality plays a crucial role in the success of any intervention. Mary's achievements experienced during our work together were strongly influenced by several aspects of her personality, including: her high level of dedication and focus to her psychological training, her task oriented style, her lack of underlying pathology, her capacity for insight, and her awareness of internal states. As she noted in one of our later sessions, psychological training takes much the same time and effort as does physical training. If athletes are to benefit from psychological interventions, they must be motivated to learn and implement the skill.

REFERENCES

Bernstein, D. A., & Borkevec, T. D. (1973). *Progressive relaxation training: A manual for helping professions.* Champaign, IL: Research Press.

Cogan, X. D., & Petrie, T. A. (1996). Consultation with college student-athletes. *College Student Journal, 30,* 9-16.

Helms, J. E. (1984). Toward a theoretical explanation of the effects of race on counseling: A black and white model. *The Counseling Psychologist, 12,* 153-164.

Linder, D. E., Pillow, D. R., & Reno, R. R. (1989). Shrinking jocks: Derogation of athletes who consult a sport psychologist. *Journal of Sport & Exercise Psychology, 11,* 270-280.

Miller, M. J., & Moore, K. X. (1993). Athletes' and nonathletes' expectations about counseling. *Journal of College Student Development, 34,* 267-269.

Morgan, W. P., Brown, D. R., Raglin, J. S., O'Connor, P. J., & Ellickson, K. A. (1987). Psychological monitoring of overtraining and staleness. *British Journal of Sports Medicine, 21,* 107-114.

Russell, R. K., Miller, D. E., & June, L. N. (1975). A comparison between group systematic desensitization and cue-controlled relaxation in the treatment of test anxiety. *Behavior Therapy. 6,* 172-177.

Taylor, J., & Schneider, B. A. (1992). The sport-clinical intake protocol: A comprehensive interviewing instrument for applied sport psychology. *Professional Psychology: Research and Practice, 23,* 318-325.

Index

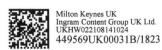